# Love Your Body Love Yourself

## the book on holistic fitness after 40

by Oprae Y.F. Park

Love Your Body Love Yourself: the book on holistic fitness after 40

Author: Oprae Y.F. Park
Cover design: Visual Arts / Janna Juan
Editor: Suzanne M. Shirley
Illustrator: Janna Juan
Exercise Demonstrator: Ramesh Koulaji
Proof Readers: Catherine Dunne, Peggy Bonnell-Prince
Layout: Janna Juan

Copyright © Oprae Y.F. Park, April 2014
ISBN: 978-0-9936766-0-4
First Edition, April 2014

*Dedicated to my mom; the kindest and strongest woman I know.*

*Also dedicated to you, my reader, who believes and trusts in your own ability to be better and is willing to do the work, even after 40.*

# Contents

## *Part III:* The Formula of Success

# Acknowledgments

My deepest love and gratitude goes:

To my wonderful parents. They not only gave me life, but also have allowed me to live and explore my own life without making judgments. As a retired nurse, my mom has been a great example for loving, caring and helping others. Since I was a little girl, I have witnessed how she helped so many people without asking anything in return. My mom and dad were always there for me no matter what happened. Dad passed away on November 18, 2012. His spirit is always around me.

To my son, Yida Li, a special gift in my life that has brought me so much joy. He keeps me humble through his constant honest feedback and comments. Thank you.

To my love, Billy Hantzakos. Thank you for allowing me to be ME, and supporting everything I do, even if it sometimes seems crazy. Knowing you has been a true blessing in my life.

To my clients who inspire me daily. They help me realize how much I love my job and how lucky and honored I am to be a part of their lives on a daily basis.

To my mentors who have had a huge influence in my personal and professional life: **Paul Chek**, the author of *How to Eat, Move and Be Healthy* and the founder of the C.H.E.K Institute in San Diego. I am so grateful for having had the opportunity to learn from Paul's work on an integrative approach to health and exercise. I've embraced it into my daily life. **Emma Lane**, the founder of Energize Mind Body, in the UK. She was my first teacher and led me down the path of holistic health and fitness. **Louise Hay**, the author of *You Can Heal Your Life* and founder of Hay House, the world's largest publishing house for personal growth. In following her work, I completely changed my beliefs about my body and my life. I am grateful.

To those who made this book possible and wonderful. Elaine Markam, who gave the title to this book; Susan Eliott, who introduced me to a young and talented artist named Janna Juan, who, through her fresh eyes, did a wonderful job on the illustrations in my book; Ramesh Koulaji, my dearest friend and holistic personal trainer who modeled for all the exercises in the book; Catherine Dunne and Peggy Prince who spent time reading chapters line by line and made the necessary corrections on my first draft.

Finally, to Rymond Aron, the New York Times best selling author, who inspired me and taught me everything I needed to know to write this book through his 10-10-10 program.

And a special acknowledgement to myself; 50 years of living on this planet has been a journey. There were so many events in my life that could have prevented me from becoming who I am and stopped me from doing what I do. I give myself huge credit for keeping an open mind, trusting my own ability to learn and grow and for being consistent. Every day I realize more and more how special and wonderful I am.

Love,

Oprae Y.F. Park

# Foreword

You can have the life, experiences, and body you want, even well beyond age 40!

Though there are many books written on the topic about being healthy at any age, there are very few written by people that have mastered their teachings in their own life. This is not the case with Oprae Park's beautiful book, Love Your Body Love Yourself: the book on holistic fitness after 40.

Oprae has been my student for several years, and I've had the joy of watching her diligently apply holistic teachings I teach in her own life. As she shares in this book, she has made several body-mind transitions. Each step of the way, Oprae discovered increased health, vitality, and freedom of self-expression. What a joy to see a book written by an author who is sharing her authentic self-experiences, as an individual, and as a skilled Holistic Lifestyle Coach!

In this outstanding book, Oprae's approach is balanced and simple and she gives very practical information that anyone can apply quickly and easily to experience rapid changes in the state of their body-mind health. She does an excellent job of integrating fundamental health essentials of how to care for your body, as well as how to use your mind to effectively create your dream life.

By reading this book, you will learn useful, easy to apply basics regarding diet and lifestyle from how to effectively eat, sleep, hydrate, mobilize your joints, stretch, and exercise with safe, intelligent progression. While most authors are confident that their books are all that's needed to make a successful life transition, Oprae is wise enough to inform her readers that one of the most important elements of a successful change process is to find a good mentor. She gives great suggestions for doing just that, and shares her own experiences of learning with skilled mentors.

### *The Life Process*

Without a doubt, the life process is complex. In fact, it is more complex today than it has ever been in human history due to a massive flood of information about pretty much everything. Though we'd naturally think that more information is a good thing, there is little evidence that "more is better" in this regard. When we look at the skyrocketing rates of disease, such as obesity and diabetes, we not only see adults suffering progressively more and more, but children too! This begs the question: "Why are we the most unhealthy people we've ever been when we have more medical doctors, therapists, nutritionists, coaches and trainers per capita than ever in history?"

As I see it, we are not suffering from a lack of opportunity to heal, grow, and live our dreams. We ARE suffering from mass confusion around issues of what is, and isn't important with regard to being healthy. We live in a culture that has been heavily influenced by corporate interests. In fact, some studies have indicated that approximately 60% of a medical doctor's education is paid for by our drug manufacturers; this is clearly a dangerous relationship when you consider that the Hippocratic Oath taken by physicians is to first do no harm. The same challenge has manifested itself in nursing, physical therapy, chiropractic, osteopathic, and the exercise profession. Almost every educational conference being run in the world today is heavily influenced by both sponsorship funding, and the content being offered.

From a professional's point of view, this is what it looks like when people become conditioned to believe in information above and beyond facts or reality. Several years ago, I was giving a lecture on holistic health principles at a large conference in New York City. While I was pointing out how dangerous sports drinks were, and exposing all the dangerous chemicals and stimulators in them, a woman raised her hand. I called on her, and with a very angry tone and scowling face, she said, "Aren't you embarrassed to be saying such things when Gatorade is the sponsor of this conference?"

I responded, informing her that I didn't personally care if Gatorade made money fall from the skies, or bought everyone's hotel rooms and meals. There is no proof like hard evidence – the body doesn't lie. Having coached countless elite athletes and people with a wide variety of illnesses and diseases back to health with natural means, I've had many chances to see how much healing takes place from removing all such commercially produced "miracle cures" from people's diets. The woman was so upset at me that she stormed out of the conference room.

The fact that people are often uninterested in seeing or hearing the truth, and that they will often defend the very ideas that are slowly killing them, is a result of what is referred to as "conditioning". Corporations with money as their driving motive have mastered "telling people what they want to hear", and not giving them what they need, nor what is promised in ads and on products. When you consider that the average person spends just under five hours a day watching TV, it becomes easy to see how their minds become conditioned to believe things that aren't true.

In my entire career, now over 30 years running, I have had a practice of helping my clients' remove all supplements and performance enhancing products, powders, drinks, pills, etc. from their diet for seven days. I have not had one single individual tell me that they didn't feel much better without them! It is very common for my clients to finish a seven day exclusion period feeling a bit confused as to why they feel so much better without all their magic pills, powders, and potions? The answer is quite simple. The grand majority of ingredients used in such miracle cures is very poor quality. They are often loaded with synthetic colors, flavors, emulsifiers, stabilizers, and use commercially farmed plant products, which are loaded with farming chemical residues. Fortunately for them, there is a better, more cost effective, environmentally friendly way to live and create our dreams together.

The systems I developed and taught Oprae and all my students through the C.H.E.K Institute are largely based on my research into developmental, or "primal humans". When we look at historical records of diseases and disease rates, we find that it was mostly acute illnesses, such as bacterial infections and environmental stress factors that limited our life span. There was very little chronic disease that plagued people, such as arthritis, heart disease, digestive/eliminative disorders, and diseases linked directly to eating poor quality food.

When you go out into the wild, you do not see overweight, out of shape, nor chronically sick animals. Have you ever seen a fat rattlesnake, coyote, or eagle in the wild? I doubt you have! And isn't it interesting that they don't watch TV, have doctors, eat processed foods, nor use medical drugs...

Oprae's book, *Love Your Body Love Yourself - the book on holistic fitness after 40,* offers the wisdom that has worked to keep us healthy for as long as people have been keeping records. In this special offering, you will learn the essentials of:

1. Having a dream worth living for, worth recreating yourself for!
2. How to eat to optimally fuel and nourish your body in your daily dream-creation process.
3. How to value and utilize rest.
4. How to correct your posture, mobilize your body, and move in ways that are nourishing to you and support your dreams each day.

Oprae also offers her beautiful Formula of Success:

A-wareness
C-ommitment
M-entor
A-ction
E-ducation, which is very in tune with my experiences as a Holistic Health Practitioner.

First and foremost, "awareness" is the key. Without awareness, we cannot effectively produce creative change in our lives; we have to be aware of what we want to become aware of what habits or behaviors no longer serve us.

When we create a dream for ourselves of our own making, we are naturally committed. That commitment inspires us to find mentors and education from masterful mentors that provides us the information we need to heal and grow. When we find the right information, which you now have, taking action becomes easy and natural.

I know you'll enjoy having Oprae as your personal mentor as much as I've enjoyed having her as my student and watching her transform herself into an authentic master. She is here to help you now, so don't delay! Lets get started on some effective dream –weaving shall we!

Love and chi,
Paul Chek

Founder, C.H.E.K Institute
Founder, PPS Success Mastery Program

# Introduction: My Journey

## *Today*

At the age of 50,

I am happy, healthy and in shape.

I have a better body shape than in my 20s and more energy than in my 30s. I am healthier than in my 40s, and most of all, I am pain free and drug free.

I believe everything is a choice and I choose to do the things that I do.

I love what I do and do what I love.

I take care of myself in every way day by day.

I say "yes" or "no" when I mean it, with love and compassion for myself and others.

I exercise regularly because I love and respect my body, not because I am afraid of either getting a disease or becoming fat.

I have no regrets for any decision I have made in my life as every experience was an opportunity that helped me to become who I really am.

I am grateful for everything I have.

However,

## My Wake Up Call Came When I Turned 40

When I turned 40 ten years ago, I looked in the mirror and saw a tired, overweight woman who was deep inside, sad and unhappy. I thought I was healthy for 18 years because I played basketball in my teens and started regular workouts in my early 20s. I religiously visited the gym 3 times a week to do group exercises. However I ate whatever I wanted, whenever I wanted. I went to bed after 1 AM almost every night. I wasn't aware of drinking water at all. From the age of 35 to 40, my stress had reached its peak after trying to settle down in Canada, being divorced and being separated from my son. At the age of 40, I weighed 148 pounds, my heaviest weight ever. I was tired and emotionally drained.

For the first time ever, I started questioning my approach to fitness and health. Am I doing the best I can for my body? Am I really healthy?

## Lost Two Best Friends Due to Cancer

Between 2001 and 2006, within 5 years, I lost two of my best friends, who were in their 40s, because of cancer. It was shocking to me as both of them had really active lifestyles. One of them was Hua Ma, my fitness role model whom I started my fitness journey with in the late 80s in Beijing, China. Losing them completely woke me up to health consciousness. I realized regular exercise does not guarantee a healthy body. There was something else missing from their lives.

## I Got Burned Out by Doing What I Love

Since I always had a passion for fitness, I became a personal trainer when I turned 40. I would get up early and go home late in order to train clients; I would miss lunch or have a late dinner because I love what I do. I even took a fitness manager position trying to do more and more. Slowly the stress was building up unknowingly. I was still training and working hard until I got a frozen shoulder in 2009. I had to leave work for one and a half years to learn and try to do everything I could to heal my right shoulder. It turned out to be one of the greatest gifts in my life. It saved me in every way.

### *Finding the Right Mentors*

There is a saying: "When a student is ready, the teacher shows up." When I was at my lowest point physically, emotionally and financially, I went on a journey with Paul Chek, the author of *How to Eat, Move and Be Healthy* and founder of the C.H.E.K institute. His holistic approach to health and exercise was the answer to my struggle. I found the root causes of my frozen shoulder, such as poor posture, the wrong breathing pattern, over-training with muscle imbalances and especially my thought patterns. For the first time ever, I was asked: "Do you love yourself?" while attending Paul's Holistic Lifestyle Coach Level 2 course. It was shocking to me that I never thought about loving myself as I was programmed to believe Self Love was selfish. I have compromised my personal needs and feelings for as long as I can remember. Because of that, I went on another journey with Louise Hay, the author of *You Can Heal Your Life* and founder of Hay House, in order to learn how to love myself. I listened to Louise Hay's audio book *101 Power Thoughts* every day for one year. I was amazed when I actually started to love my body and love myself every day, everything else became easier and easier. My body and my life gave me back what I really wanted, effortlessly.

## A Brief List of What I have Changed in 10 Years

| Habits | Old | New |
|---|---|---|
| Thinking | » I don't deserve.<br>» My legs are too short.<br>» I need approval for my decisions. | » I deserve the best.<br>» I have a perfect body.<br>» I love and approve of myself. |
| Breathing | » Not aware of it at all.<br>» Mouth breathing most of the time. I snored a lot when sleeping. | » Conscious abdominal breathing throughout the day.<br>» Nose breathing most of the time. When sleeping, I'm quiet and peaceful. |
| Sleeping | » Always went to bed after 1:00 AM.<br>» Woke up tired most of the time. | » Go to bed before 10:30 PM.<br>» Wake up alert and energetic. |
| Diet | » No breakfast<br>» Only 2-3 glasses of water daily<br>» 3 cups of coffee with triple sugar daily<br>» Processed food, such as orange juice and frozen dinner<br>» Low fat, high starchy food<br>» Whole wheat bread every day | » Always have breakfast.<br>» 2.5 L of clean water daily<br>» One single espresso daily, no sugar<br>» Whole, local organic food<br>» High protein/fat, low starchy food<br>» Wheat and gluten free |
| Movement | » Cardio classes all the time<br>» No regular stretches<br>» No weight training<br>» Tai Chi, yoga or Qi Gong were not my thing | » No more than 20 minutes of cardio<br>» Regular stretching and corrective exercises<br>» Weight lifting<br>» Tai Chi and Qi Gong regularly |

## *What does Holistic Fitness Mean to Me*

Holistic Fitness to me is about balancing every aspect of life on a day-to-day basis. It includes mental/emotional/spiritual balance, nutrition/lifestyle balance, physical balance, social balance, work balance and financial balance. Each component is just as important as the others, like puzzle pieces are for the whole picture.

**Mental/emotional/spiritual balance** has to do with my 10 minutes of daily breathing and meditation that raises my awareness, of observing my thoughts without judgment, being able to consciously choose loving and supportive thoughts, and being willing to forgive myself and others. It also has to do with experiencing a sense of purpose, of belonging and feeling alive every day. It is about fulfilling a life which is aligned with what I love and care about the most. It allows me to live in the present moment.

**Nutrition/lifestyle balance** is about feeding my body 3 - 4 times a day with nutrient dense whole foods and at all costs; it must be free of toxins. It is about letting my body guide me on the best macronutrient ratio (vegetables vs. protein and healthy fat) for optimum energy and mental focus. It is also about drinking 2.5 liters of clean water daily no matter how busy I am, going to bed by 10:30 PM most nights, and identifying the source of any stress and managing it in every way I can.

**Physical balance** has to do with choosing the right type of activity/movement I need the most, based on the energy level I have and then creating a realistic plan to fit it into my daily life. It could be 5 minutes of mobilizing/stretching, or 15 - 30 minutes of circuit movements. The more workload I have in a day, the shorter the workout I will have as I need to balance my energy.

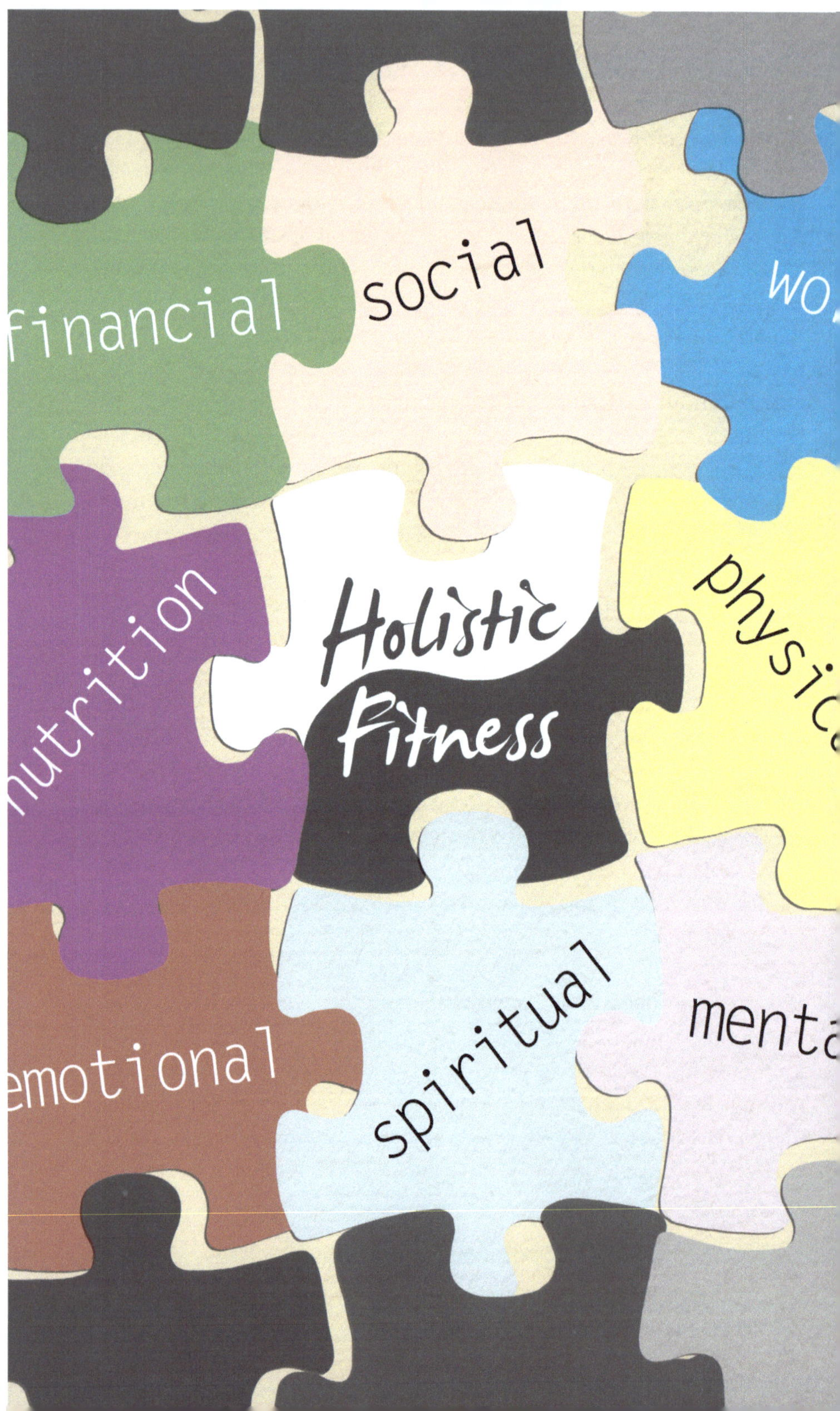
financial
social
wo
nutrition
Holistic Fitness
physic
spiritual
menta
emotional

**Social balance** is about surrounding myself with people who bring out the best in me, those who leave me feeling energized rather than depleted. In addition, being true to my values in everything I do in life and respecting other people's values and choices with compassion.

**Work balance** has to do with having a work schedule that supports my body's rhythm in terms of how much stress it can handle and how much time it needs to recharge my energy in order to have the most productive day without depleting my body. By the end of the day, I make sure I still have 20% of my energy left so that I can do other activities like grocery shopping, being with loved ones and feeding my body with a healthy dinner. For example, I won't take a 6 o'clock client in the morning; I always leave work for 30 minutes to have lunch at a quiet place and I chew my food with gratitude; I won't take clients in the late evening; I keep my daily limit at six clients.

**Financial balance** is about taking care of my financial freedom and taking action on financial education, maintaining healthy spending habits, managing debt and keeping a close eye on personal investments. I believe it is our birthright to have a healthy, happy body and have financial freedom. Anything can be learned.

## My Holistic Fitness Pyramid

Based on what I have learned and practiced for a decade, I developed my holistic fitness pyramid as on the next page. In this book, I will share with you step by step how to build this holistic pyramid to achieve happiness, health and a perfect body. If it makes sense to you, pick this book and work on it. If I can do it after 40, so can you!

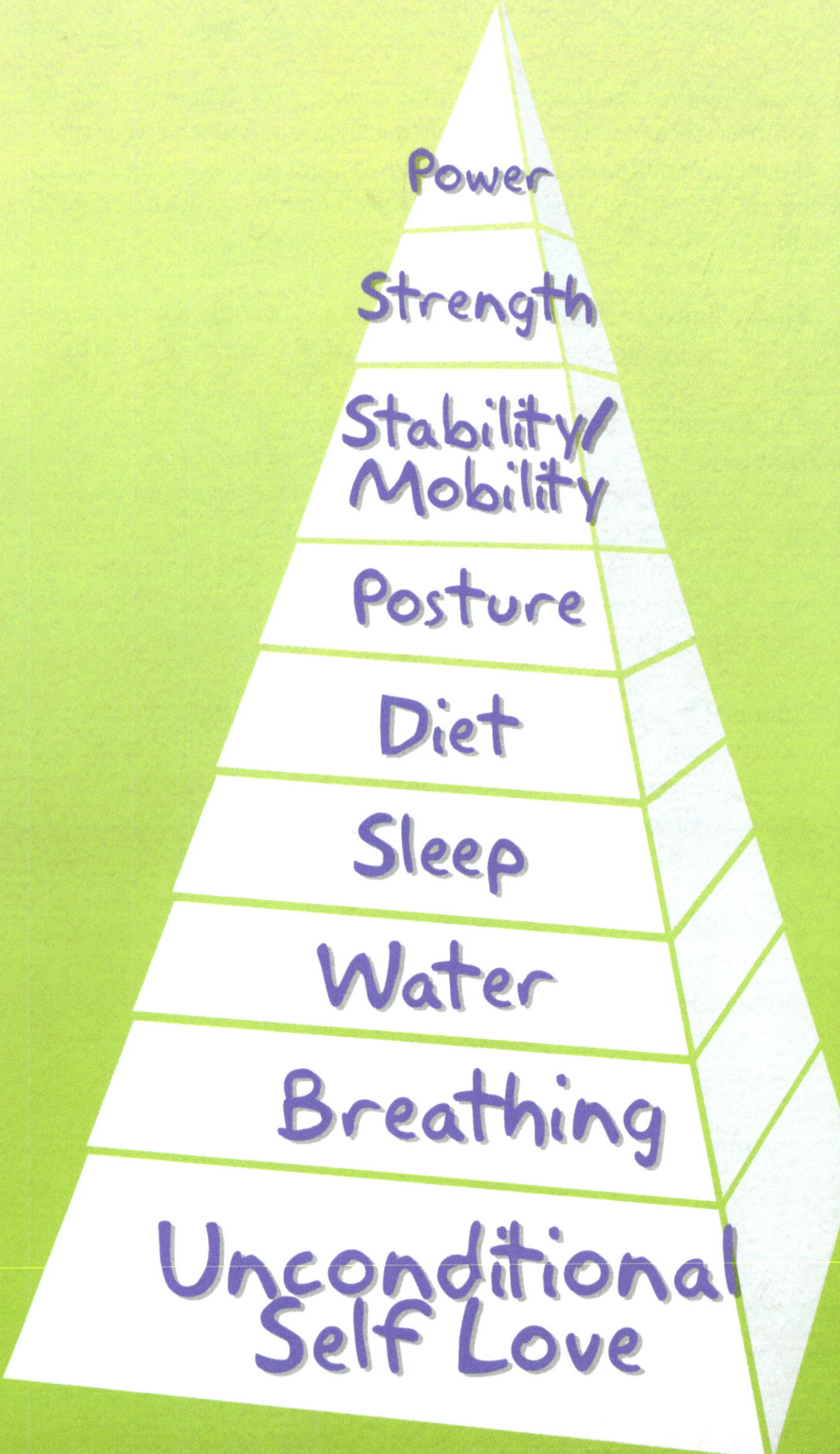
Power
Strength
Stability/
Mobility
Posture
Diet
Sleep
Water
Breathing
Unconditional
Self Love

# *Part I*

# Foundation of Holistic Fitness After 40

*If you are over 40, and have started getting symptoms, such as gaining weight, chronic fatigue, depression, high blood pressure, chronic joint inflammation, poor digestion and poor sleep quality, what is on your mind? More exercise or a healthier diet? Have you thought that maybe all of those symptoms were not just brought on by a lack of exercise or the wrong diet but rather caused by an imbalance from a combination of factors? You very well may be out of balance in terms of your thought pattern, breathing pattern, eating pattern, sleeping pattern and movement pattern. Holistic fitness after 40 is not about more diet or exercise. It is about looking inside and being aware of which pattern(s) may be blocking the way to your success. Without consciously changing those habits or patterns, no exercise or pill can restore you.*

## Balance Energy and Health First

*Energy is simply a life force. It is essential to health, well-being and fitness. Everything we do and every choice we make has an impact on our energy level. For example: when working, playing, creating, exercising, cooking and shopping, we spend energy; while drinking water, eating food, sleeping, and breathing fully we help create or reserve energy.*

*Unfortunately most of us are experts at spending energy but poor managers when it comes to reserving energy. Often I see people over 40 making a big commitment to exercise and eat well, but they barely have enough energy to carry them through their daily work and do activities like shopping and preparing healthy food. Yet I see them wasting so much energy on thinking stressful thoughts, shallow breathing, not drinking enough clean water, and not having enough sleep... The body doesn't lie. Without energy you will have a compromised immune system, poor digestion and a dysfunctional hormone system, making fitness impossible to achieve and maintain.*

*No matter what your goal is - losing weight, having more energy, eliminating pain, or having a nicely toned body, the first thing to do is to build a foundation - Energy and Health. It is like building a house, the stronger the foundation, the more solid and long lasting the house.*

*As much as I have loved exercise, I strongly believe that we must address and build fundamental daily habits on thinking, breathing, water, sleep and individualized diet that can restore energy and health. After age 40, we need to work smarter not harder.*

*In the next five chapters, I am going to share with you the things you can do to dramatically improve your energy and vitality every day by thinking right, breathing right, drinking right, eating right and sleeping right. Once you get those things in place, your body will have plenty of energy for exercise. You will be so pumped. Believe me.*

BREATHE
WATER
REST
DIET
STRETCH
SUPPORTIVE
THOUGHTS

*Balanced Energy*

WORK
PLAY
SHOP
COOK
EXERCISE
CREATE

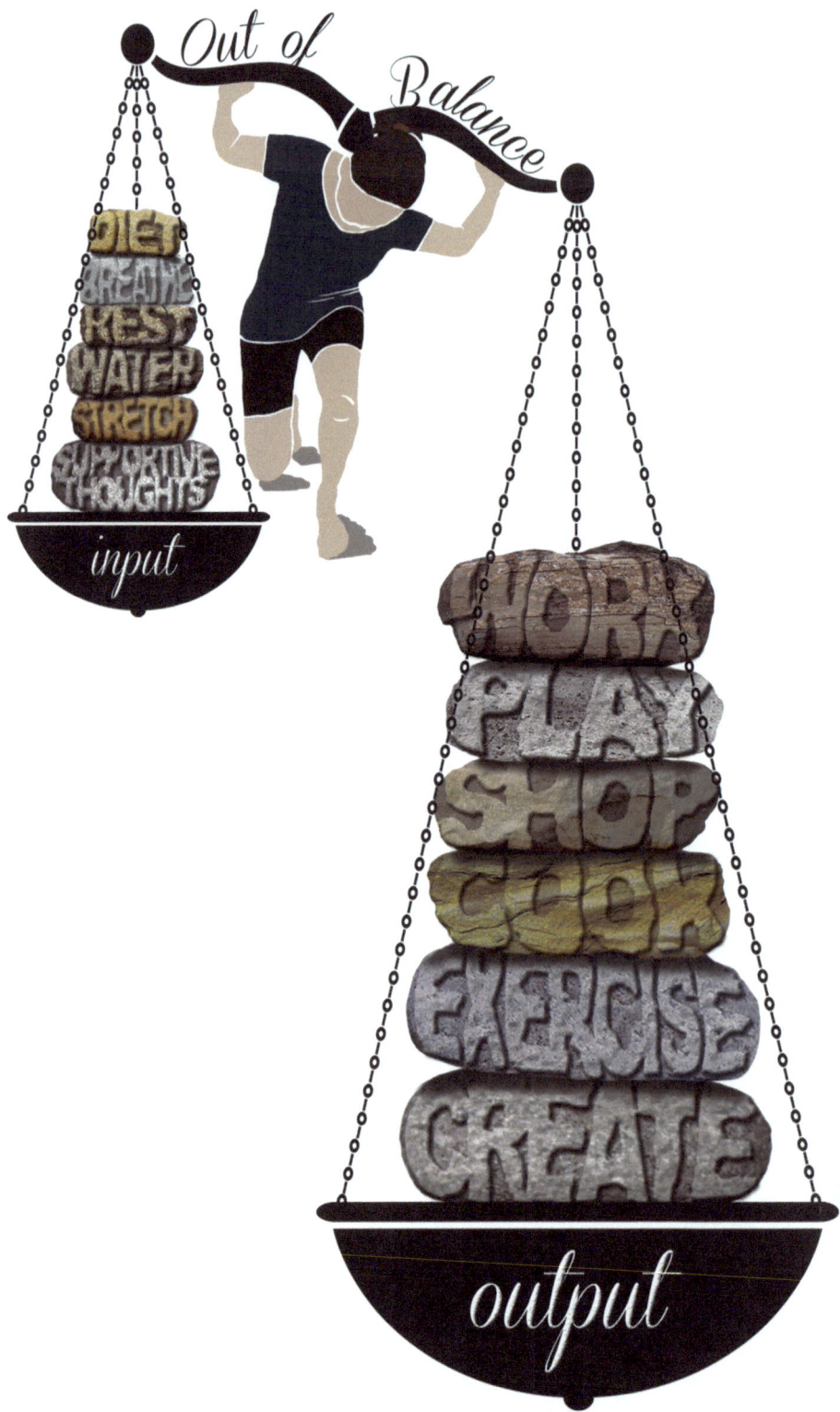

Out of Balance

input

WORK
PLAY
SHOP
COOK
EXERCISE
CREATE

output

I have a perfect body.

I am grateful for the body and health I have now.

Everything is a choice; I choose to be healthy, happy and fit.

I deserve to be healthy and happy.

I love, trust and approve of myself.

I always take care of myself first.

I am lighter and freer everyday.

It is easy to make a change.

# DAILY
## AFFIRMATIONS
### *for a*
# PERFECT BODY

# 1

## *Change Your Thoughts, Change Your Body*

*"We cannot solve our problems with the same
thinking we used when we created them."*
*- Albert Einstein*

................................................

Every thought you think, every decision you make creates your
physical experience and forms your body. The same thoughts you
had yesterday towards your body, life, food, and exercise form the
life and body you have today. We are the creators of our bodies and
our lives. Just being aware of it gives us the power to change.

### *Every Thought Has Energy and Emotion Attached to It*

Everything starts with a thought. We are said to have 50,000 - 68,000
thoughts a day. They have a powerful impact on our cells, organs,
hormones, breathing pattern and more. The human brain uses up to
30% of our energy daily. Do these thoughts sound familiar?

» I am tired.
» I'll never lose weight.
» It is hard to build muscles.
» It is horrible.
» I am not good enough.
» I am weak.
» My life sucks.

Guess what? Your body believes every word you say. You are what
you think.

..............................................

Do you fight with yourself mentally every day with negative thinking, or do you work to align your thoughts with what you truly intend for your body and your life?

..............................................

## *Different Emotions Affect Different Organs*

Chinese medicine discovered thousands of years ago the relationship between emotions and the influence they have on our organs. They discovered that anger, frustration and jealousy disrupt liver and gall bladder functions, such as the production of more cholesterol, an imbalance in bile production, and a diminished ability to detoxify the body. Fear weakens the kidneys and bladder, leading to a loss of sexual energy and life force, plus nervous system disorders. Sadness and depression affect lungs and the large intestine, seen as a breathing problem and constipation. Worry, anxiety and mistrust interfere with the stomach, spleen and pancreas, which cause poor digestion and insulin mismanagement. Hate or impatience influences the heart and small intestine, which causes high blood pressure or chest pain.

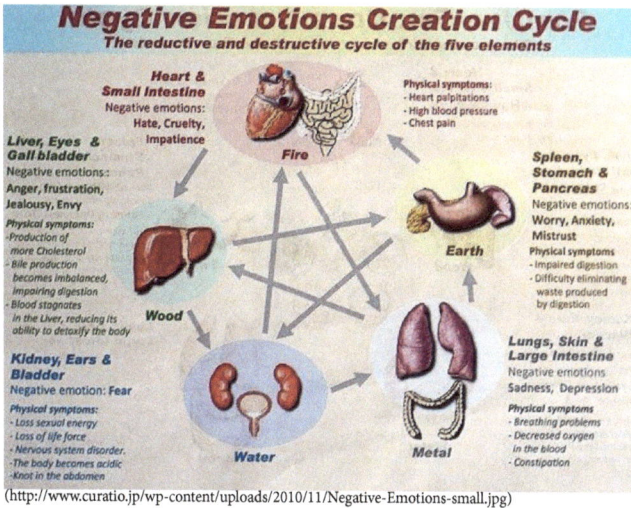

(http://www.curatio.jp/wp-content/uploads/2010/11/Negative-Emotions-small.jpg)

## Reprogram Your Thoughts

*"Your body is merely a screen onto which is projected the
nature of your thoughts. When the weight is gone from your
consciousness, it will be gone from your physical experience."*
*- Marianne Williamson, author of*
*"A Course of Miracle in Weight Loss"*

·············································

According to Bruce Lipton, the author of *Biology of Beliefs*, we are living with both a conscious mind and a subconscious mind. Conscious mind is the creative mind that holds our wishes, desires, commitments and positive thinking. In contrast, the subconscious mind is the habitual mind that takes care of most of our daily choices. Neuroscience has shown that 95% of our life experience is run by our subconscious mind.

The subconscious mind is formed by what we saw, heard and experienced over and over when we grew up, especially before the age of seven. Unfortunately the beliefs stored in our subconscious mind about ourselves and our bodies are not consciously chosen by us. Most of them are from parents, society, teachers or friends. Now we have the opportunity to replace them with ones that support our life and body.

When you choose thoughts consciously that are aligned with the body and life you are intended to have, you already have chosen the body and life that manifests those thoughts. It is like you plant seeds in the field, when you water and nourish them every day, they will grow and bloom. Be very careful when you think or say "I AM". If you think or say "I am tired", or "I am useless", every cell in your body hears it. Your 100 trillion cells don't just hear it they react to it, hormonally and functionally. If a thought makes you angry, depressed, or sad, replace it with something like "I am energetic", "I am loved".

## 1. Turn down all noise

*"If you want to be full, you have to be empty first."*
*- Tao masters*

In order to let new ideas and new ways of thinking to start working for you, the best way is to consciously choose what you hear, see and experience every day. Don't let fear-based news and emotions or the ideas of others take control of yours. For example, if you keep watching *The Biggest Loser* every week, you may adopt the belief that you need to beat yourself up to lose weight and you will end up doing a crazy work out that might even hurt you. If a drug commercial pops up every 3 minutes telling you it will help your lower back pain, it is very likely you will subconsciously choose that drug when you encounter lower back pain. All commercials are designed to program your subconscious beliefs without you taking notice.

Every morning when I turn on my computer and open my mail box, the first thing I do is to delete all the junk emails or any email that doesn't interest me. I read less than 10% of the emails I get daily. The same thing applies with my mind. I only allow those thoughts that support my body and lifestyle, such as "I am healthy", "I am energetic", and "I have the perfect body." instead of "I am sick", "I am tired", and "I don't have a nice body". Remember, "No thought stays in your head rent free".

I haven't watched news on TV nor listened to the radio in years. I only choose the topics that I am interested in when I listen and watch. I listen to conference recordings which are related to personal development, or lectures on nutrition, exercises, or interviews that uplift me. I save my energy and time for what I need the most.

## 2. Surround yourself with positive friends

Having a supportive social circle is very important. People are naturally resistant to changing because it is more comfortable living with their old habits. It is very likely that when you start to change, friends and family around you who are afraid of changing will tell you their stories and offer their opinions. It is okay for them to think that way. But now you don't have the same interests or purpose in life anymore, so you have to let them go. Once you let old influences disappear you are going to attract people along your journey who have the same purpose as you.

## 3. Daily intentional thoughts/affirmations

One of the most well-known mentors and teachers in the world for affirmations is Louise Hay, the author of *You Can Heal Your Life* and founder of Hay House, the largest publishing company on personal growth. In 2009, my life was at its lowest point emotionally, physically and financially. I had to quit my job because of a frozen shoulder caused by over-training, emotional and work related stress. A friend gave me Louise Hay's audio book *101 Power Thoughts*. It caught my attention right away. It was like something I had waited all my life to hear. I started to listen to it every day. Actually, I listened to it for a whole year every morning while I was cooking. It calmed my mind by taking me to a place without self-judgment, regret or resentment. Slowly those affirmations I needed the most became a part of my subconscious belief system.

Whenever I find myself in a stressful situation those affirmations return to my consciousness. For example, when I am in a rush, I start telling myself "I have all the time in the world, time stretches when I need it". When I make a mistake, I always think "Every experience is an opportunity to learn and grow. I am safe". When I feel neck and shoulder pain I gently say "I love every inch of my body inside and out". Intentional thoughts or daily affirmations reset the subconscious mind for success. It is easy to do and very effective.

Read the following intentional thoughts or affirmations and feel the ones that you agree with the most:

- » I love, trust and approve of myself.
- » Everything is a choice. I choose to be healthy, happy and fit.
- » I am grateful for the body and health I have now.
- » I create a healthier happier body with every breath I take.
- » I deserve to be healthy and happy.
- » I have a perfect body.
- » I am lighter and freer every day.
- » It is easy to make a change.
- » I always have time for eating healthy and exercising.
- » Water is essential to my life, I enjoy drinking clean water throughout the day.
- » I have all the energy and vitality I need for all the things I love to do.
- » Every day in every way I make healthy choices.
- » It is easy to listen to my body's messages and take appropriate action.
- » I trust my body's wisdom. All my cells, organs, muscles and joints are supporting my health and fitness.
- » I always take care of myself first.
- » I love and nurture my body every day.
- » Each day I send my body positive, supportive and loving messages.
- » I deserve to have the body and life I love.

*8 Steps to Love Your Body, Love Yourself Unconditionally*

Think about this, who in the entire world has the longest relationship with you? I am sure you know the answer. Yes it's YOU. Love is the center of your being. Practice unconditional love for yourself daily, stop fighting with yourself. Accept who you are and take small steps, one at a time. When you truly love yourself and your body, you will make better choices on breathing, food, water, sleep and exercise; you will be under less stress and will not be fearful of failing and of the disapproval of others; you will be truly inspired to get well and get in shape; you will have a sense of self-acceptance and self-approval. Self-love is the essence of holistic fitness.

Please take the following 8 steps to love your body, love yourself:

## 1. Stop criticizing yourself

Be gentle with yourself. Criticism doesn't change anything, nor motivate you to do better. Accept yourself exactly as who you are at this moment. By doing so it helps renew your energy and helps you make better choices in the next moment. Every minute the old you dies, the new you is reborn. You have the power to choose what you can do now. Please don't give away your power.

## 2. Forgive yourself

Forgiveness will set you free. Know that you did the best you could at that time with the awareness, understanding, and knowledge you had then. So did others. The past is over and done. Let it go. You are changing and growing. So are others. Even just the willingness to forgive will take the emotional stress off your shoulders and make you feel lighter and freer.

## 3. Take care of yourself first

You cannot truly take care of others unless you take care of yourself first. As my mentor Paul Chek said "You cannot give what you don't have". This is extremely important for women over 40 since we always put ourselves after our family's needs, our work place's demands and friends' requests. With this habit of over-giving I burned myself out, and more women than I can count have done exactly the same thing.

Learn to say "no" with deep love and compassion for yourself and without feeling guilty. One of the best authorities on self-care is Cheryl Richardson, the author of *The Art of Extreme Self Care*. I was laughing and crying when I read her book the first time. I remembered there was a chapter called Let Me Disappoint You. It gave me the courage to step out of my old life which was full of compromises and sacrifices.

## 4. Always find a way to praise yourself

Every morning when I wake up, I always say to myself "Oprae, I love you. You are my hero". It makes me feel like I am important and loved. It also gives me the energy to get out of bed and do what I am supposed to do. During the day I always find a way to praise myself like I'll say, "Oprae, you did such a good job making a nutritional breakfast for yourself and the family", "Well done for stretching for 10 minutes today".

Say to yourself that you are doing a good job when you drink a cup of clean water first thing in the morning. Thank yourself that you are taking a healthy lunch to work, or take a short walk after dinner. By the end of the day, don't forget to say "Good job, buddy, we made it through the day. I am grateful for what I did today".

## 5. Focus only on what you can, not what you can't

"What you focus on expands." If you focus on problems, they tend to become bigger. On the other hand, if you focus on what you can do, it is very likely that you will do things right. Several years ago when I had a busy day with 6 or 7 clients, I often became stressed with the thought that I didn't have a full hour to exercise. It just added more stress to what I already had. Now when I am in the same situation I always make sure that I am eating extremely well and drinking enough water, plus I make sure I have a good sleep the night before. Then I go with 10 - 15 minutes of stretching or do some Tai Chi to restore enough energy to meet my workload. I don't stress my body by forcing it to over spend its energy.

## 6. Be patient

Acknowledge that you are in the process of changing. Dream big, start with a small step and keep doing small things every day. Never chase the results. Just do the right thing, and let the results come to you. Building a new habit takes time. A thousand miles is accomplished by taking every single step. Be happy that you are on the right path. And tell yourself that you are closer to becoming who you really are day by day.

## 7. Be grateful

Before going to sleep, take a moment to take 10 deep breaths and think of three things you are grateful for. It doesn't matter how small or big they are. Think things like: "I am grateful that I did 5 minutes of breathing this morning", "I am grateful for beautiful weather today", or "I am grateful for being with my loved one tonight".

## 8. Have fun

Find something fun and enjoyable and do it on a regular basis. Life is about enjoyment and creativity. Children are masters of playing and creating. They are our teachers. My son's daily workout is dancing with the music he loves, then push-ups and abs. It motivates him and he does it every day without feeling bored.

Since I was a little girl I loved to dance but I was intimated by my inflexibility and the complicated choreography. Inspired by Misty Tripoli's Unite and Unique dance philosophy I recently took TheGroove facilitator training to fulfill my childhood dream (www. theworldgroovemovement.com). Instead of going on the treadmill for a cardio workout, I am having so much fun grooving. Meeting my friends for lunch or coffee on a regular basis also makes me happy and keeps me fulfilled.

Give yourself a permission to find something you love and do it often.

---

#### Take Action

*Intentional thought: "I love my body, I love myself."*

1. Every morning before you get up, be aware of what you think first. Fill your mind with intentional thoughts like: "Today is a great day," "I always have time to exercise," "I love my body," "Life loves me."

2. Write down your own intentional thoughts or affirmations on a piece of paper in color and put it on your kitchen cabinet, or bathroom wall. Read them aloud to yourself once a day for the next 6 weeks and see what will happen.

3. Before you go to sleep every night, take few deep breaths and think of three things or people you are grateful for. Make it a habit.

---

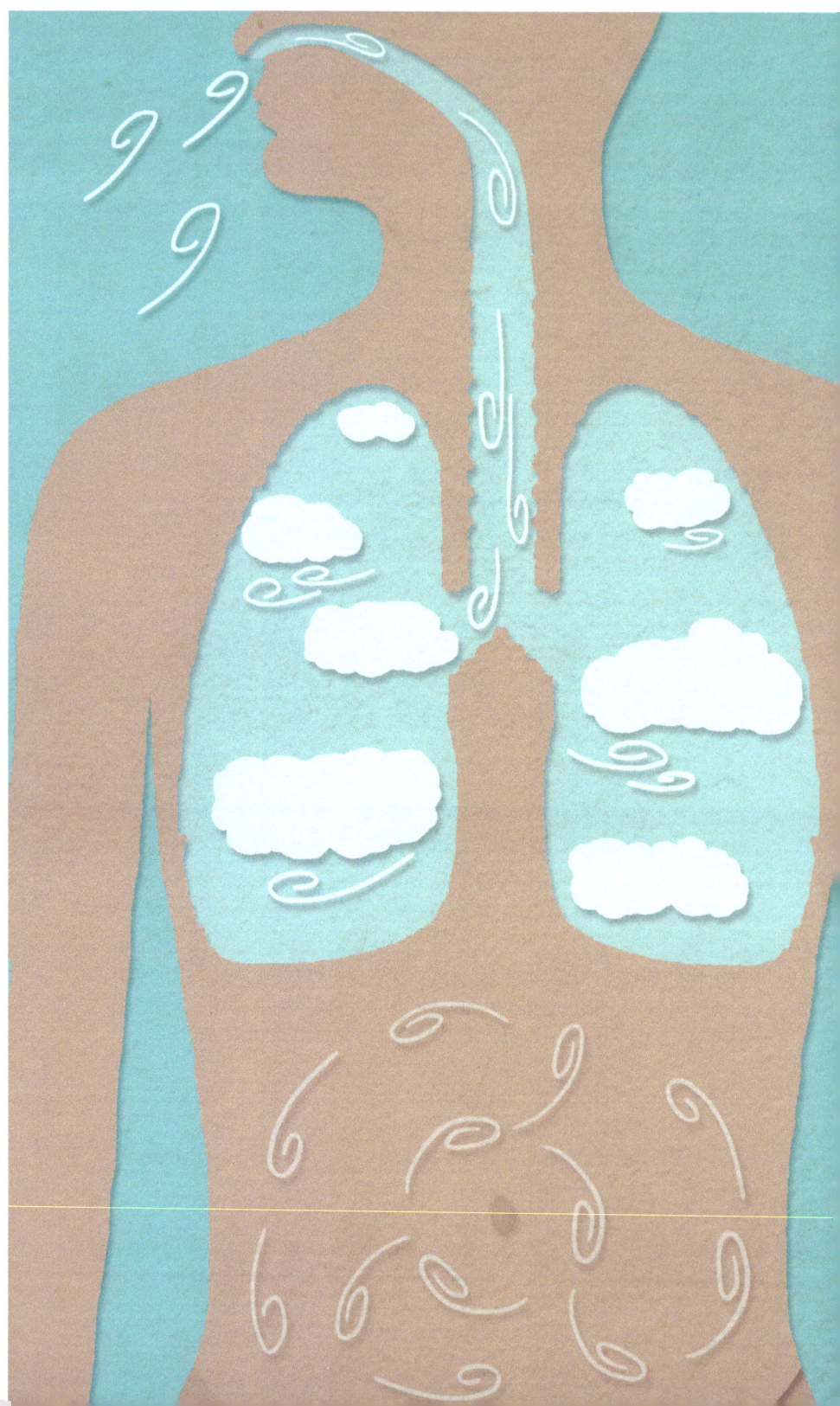

# 2

## *The Secret to Having Energy*

*"To breathe is to live. To breathe fully is to live fully,
to manifest the full range and power of our inborn potential
for vitality in everything that we sense, feel, think and do."
- Dennis Lewis, author of "The Tao of Natural Breathing"*

........................................

### *Do You Feel Tired for No Reason?*

You know you need to go to the gym to workout but you just have
no motivation and energy at all. Or you have to have a cup of coffee
and a sugary snack to pick you up. It is common to see people over
40 complaining about having low energy. Statistics shows that about
66% of the entire population has indications of adrenal fatigue syndrome, such as:

» Feeling tired for no reason.
» Have trouble getting up in the morning.
» Feeling rundown or overwhelmed.
» Have difficulty bouncing back from stress or illness.
» Have a hard time recovering from exercise.
» Crave salty and sweet snacks.
» Feel more awake, alert and energetic after 6:00 PM than you do
  all day.
» Low sex drive.

## Where Stress Comes From

Knowingly or unknowingly, our stress comes from these six sources:

**Physical stress**: from pain, lack of sleep, no exercise or over-training.

**Mental/Emotional/Spiritual stress:** from being with an abusive partner or boss, compromising your personality to please others, negative thoughts toward your body and life, or having no purpose in life.

**Chemical stress:** from consuming food sprayed with pesticides and herbicides, drinking tap water, or using personal care and home cleaning products that contain a variety of harmful chemicals.

**Nutritional stress:** from going too long without eating, chronic dehydration, or not eating the right ratio of protein, carbohydrate and fat.

**Electromagnetic stress:** from an over use of cell phones, computers and a high definition TV.

**Thermal stress:** from being in an environment which is too hot or too cold.

According to the American Academy of Family Physicians, two-thirds of all office visits to family physicians are due to stress related symptoms.

........................................

*"Stress is linked to six leading causes of death - heart disease,
cancer, lung ailments, accidents, cirrhosis of the liver, and suicide."
- Lyle H. Miller, Ph.D. and Alma Dell Smith, Ph.D.,
"The Stress Solution: An Active Plan to Manage the Stress in Your Life"*

## Fight or Flight Response

All stress adds up. Your body activates its sympathetic nervous system to deal with stress. It creates a fight or flight response, like your body's 911 system. The adrenal glands mobilize your body's response to every kind of stress in life through hormones like adrenaline and cortisol which regulate blood sugar mobilization, energy production and storage, heart rate, breathing rate, muscle tone and many other responses that help you to cope with stress.

After a stressful event, stress hormone cortisol is supposed to go back to its normal level. But if you have ongoing stress, one follows the other, the adrenal glands cannot keep up the work. As a result, every function in your body is profoundly affected. For example, your carbohydrate, protein and fat metabolism, fluid and electrolyte balance, heart and cardiovascular system, digestion and detoxification system, even your sex drive are all compromised by stress.

Energy is everything. Managing the flow of energy moment by moment is a MUST if you want to be healthy, lose weight, build muscles, and achieve better performance. I always say to my clients: "It is not in the body's best interests to lose weight or build muscles if it is under stress all the time."

Simply,

**Low energy = Survival mode = Fat storage**

## *A Big Energy Drain*

## Self-Check Your Breathing Pattern

Stand in front of a mirror, put one hand on your chest, another on your belly button. Bend your knees slightly. Relax your neck, shoulders and your entire body. Breathe in and out and observe your body.

When you inhale, is your belly rising first, or is it your chest? Are your shoulders moving? Are you using your mouth or nose?

When you exhale, does your belly flatten first, or does your chest? Are your shoulders moving? Are you using your mouth or your nose?

Chest breathing and mouth breathing are the most common breathing patterns for people who are under chronic stress. Occasionally I see clients with an inverse breathing pattern, meaning the belly flattens when inhaling and rises when exhaling. Later on I will share with you some healthy breathing tips.

**Self-Check Your Breathing Rate**

Use a watch or the timer on your iPhone. Remain still in a comfortable position. Count how many breaths (breathing in and out) you take in 60 seconds. Write it down on a piece of paper.

At rest, we should take 8-12 breaths per minute with 4-6 liters of air.

Let's use 10 breaths per minute as an optimal breathing rate. If your breathing rate is 10 or lower, congratulations. If your breathing rate is over 10, use that number minus 10 and multiply by 1440 (that is total minutes in a day: 60 minutes x 24 = 1440 minutes). I hope you are not surprised by the number. For example: one of my clients breathes 20 times per minute:

$(20-10) \times 1440 = 14,400$

Imagine how much energy the body has to use to take 14,400 extra breaths. No wonder a lot of people are tired for no apparent reason.

**Chronic Breathing Dysfunction May Be Associated with:**

» Low energy and high stress. The lungs can use only one-third of their capacity if the breathing pattern is wrong. It is important to know that 70 percent of the body's waste products are eliminated through the lungs, while the rest are eliminated through urine and feces.
» Muscle stiffness around the neck, shoulder and chest areas.
» An acid/alkaline imbalance, making the body more acidic.
» A reduced amount of digestive juices, including the enzyme pepsin, which is necessary for proper digestion.
» Constipation as shallow breathing slows down the process of peristalsis in the small and large intestines, which causes toxins to pile up and fester throughout the digestive tract.
» Weight gain.

...............................................

*"In short, such breathing weakens and disharmonizes the functioning of almost every major system in the body and makes us more susceptible to chronic and acute illness and 'dis-eases' of all kind: infections, constipation, respiratory illnesses, digestive problems, ulcers, depression, sexual disorders, sleep disorders, fatigue, headaches, poor bloodcirculation, premature aging, and so on. Many researchers even believe that our bad breathing habits also contribute to life-threatening diseases such as cancer and heart disease."*
*- Dennis Lewis, author of "The Tao of Natural Breathing"*

## *The Secret of Energy*

Breathing is something given by nature at birth. Babies have beautiful breathing rhythms by raising their bellies up and down. A full breath activates the parasympathetic branch of the autonomic nervous system, which is responsible for relaxation, digestion, detoxification, and regeneration.

Unfortunately with constant stress and poor posture over the years, most people over 40 have lost the ability to breathe fully. I have been doing a breathing assessment with every new client that comes to me. I find 100% of them have the wrong breathing pattern, such as chest breathing. That is shocking!

The more I study, practice and observe my clients, the more I value the energy flow created by every full breath. If we don't breath for 5 minutes, the brain may go into a coma. It is that simple.

**Restoring Your Breathing Pattern Can Be a Game Changer**

Breathing fully improves your energy level by increasing the circulation of blood and lymphatic fluids. It also balances the PH level in the blood, and helps you lose weight, build muscles, and perform at optimal levels.

Breathing is a powerful tool given by nature to enhance our energy and health. When you breathe fully moment by moment, you will enjoy the energy flow created within effortlessly, the inner wisdom brought into your consciousness, the unlimited connection between you and the consciousness of the universe, and the healing processes occurring on cellular level. All this can be achieved by breathing fully and consciously.

When healthy breathing is restored, energy production is much improved, the metabolism of food and the elimination of waste are more efficient; any inflammation is healed more quickly; mental clarity and focus are present. If you are overweight a reduction of weight may occur, whereas if you are underweight your weight may normalize.

For me, practicing my breathing every day is not just for mental focus and spirituality, it is also for restoring energy and health, as well as for achieving optimal physical performance. Now I understand why Tao masters are saying: "achieving things by doing nothing".

## Breathing Tips

Several times a day, check how you breathe and practice the following:

### 1. Breathe through your nose

At rest, breathing should be soft and silent, through the nose. The nose helps to regulate the volume of air we breathe. It cleans, warms and humidifies the air preparing it for the lungs. Breathing through the nose also tells the body to relax. You should feel easy, comfortable, revitalized, and refreshed. You should also feel a relaxation in the neck, shoulders and upper chest. For someone not in the habit of nose breathing, it may take time to learn how. Keep trying until it becomes second nature to you.

### 2. Breathe using your abdomen

The primary breathing muscles are the diaphragm, abdominal wall and pelvic floor. The main movement of breathing is felt deeply within the lower torso (70%-80%) and less movement is felt in the upper torso (20%-30%). This is why we are told to practice abdominal breathing. If you put one hand on your belly button and the other on your chest, you should feel the lower hand rising when breathing in and falling when breathing out. The other hand on your chest is not rising until the last one-third of each breath. Think about filling a balloon with air when breathing in. This can help you do it more easily. Correct abdominal breathing is three dimensional.

### 3. Relax when breathing

When you relax your shoulders, neck and whole body, your body knows how to breathe correctly. Do not force your breathing or think too much about any breathing technique. Just trust the body. You are born a breathing master.

## 4. Breathe with good posture

Without good posture, it is hard to breathe deeply and effectively. Someone with forward head posture tends to breathe through his/her mouth or to have shallow chest breathing. By holding your chin in and keeping your head in alignment with the upper spine, you will find it is easier to breathe deeply.

## *Breathing Exercises*

(Love Your Body, Love Yourself Exercise DVD, in which you can find all exercises in this book will be available at www.amazon.com and www.wisdomfitbyoprae.com soon.)

### 1. Qi Gong Breathing

**Set up:**
» Stand with feet apart about shoulder-width, knees slightly bent, shoulders relaxed.

**Start:**
» Gently raise both arms in front of your chest with palms facing each other, and arms close to each other, imagining you are holding a small ball.
» Breathe in while opening your arms in front of your chest, imagining you are making the ball larger.
» Breathe out and move your arms close to each other with your palms facing each other.

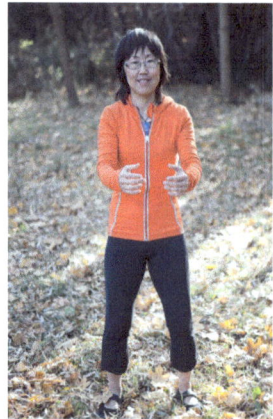

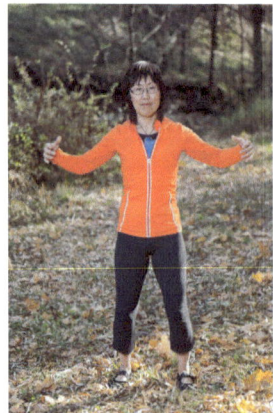

## 2. Tai Chi Ruler

**Set up:**
- » Stand with one foot 45 degrees forward.
- » Naturally drop your hands in front of your thighs with palms facing each other.

**Start:**
- » Inhale and move 70% of your body weight forward onto your front foot without raising your body. At the same time slowly raise both your arms up until your hands are on top of your head.
- » Exhale, and move 70% of your body weight backward onto your rear foot while slowly moving your arms down.
- » Do 15 - 20 times, or as many as you like. Then switch, putting the other foot forward and repeat the moves.

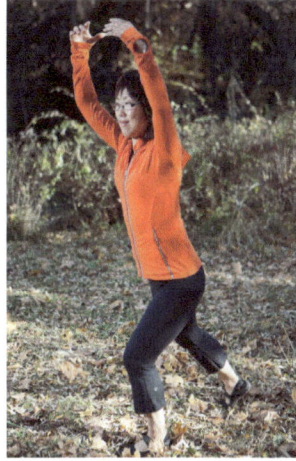

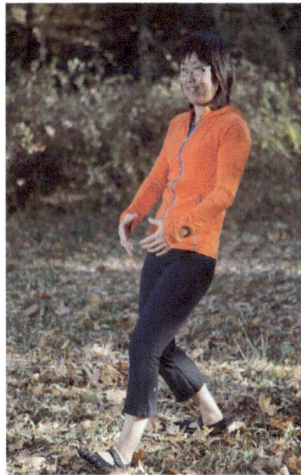

## 3. Breathing Squat

### Set up:
» Stand with feet open wider than your shoulders. Your arms are relaxed at your sides.

### Start:
» Inhale, then exhale and move your hips down and back as if you are sitting on a chair. Inhale as you return to standing position.
» Repeat at the same pace that you naturally breathe. Breathe through your nose.

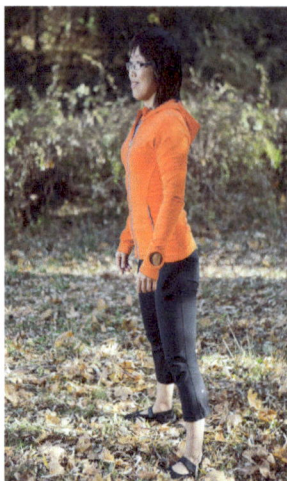

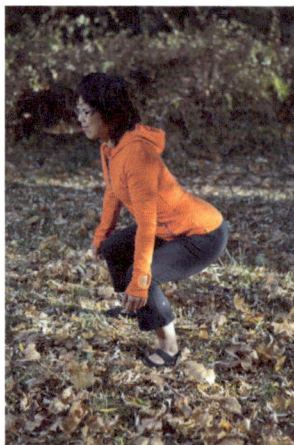

······Take Action······

*Intentional thought: "I am healthier and happier with every breath I take."*

1. Watch the free breathing exercise video at www.wisdomfitbyoprae. com.

2. Do 5-10 minutes of breathing exercises every morning or evening.

3. Several times of the day, check your breathing when you are driving or under a high stress level. Consciously practice healthy breathing for a couple of minutes or longer.

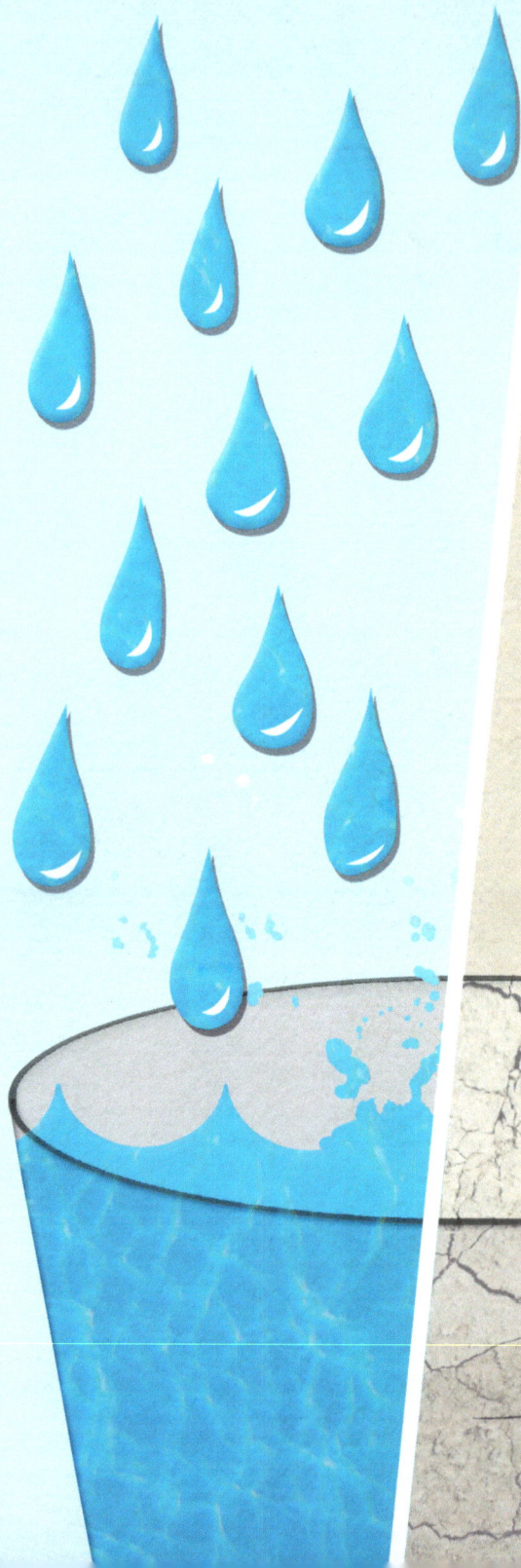

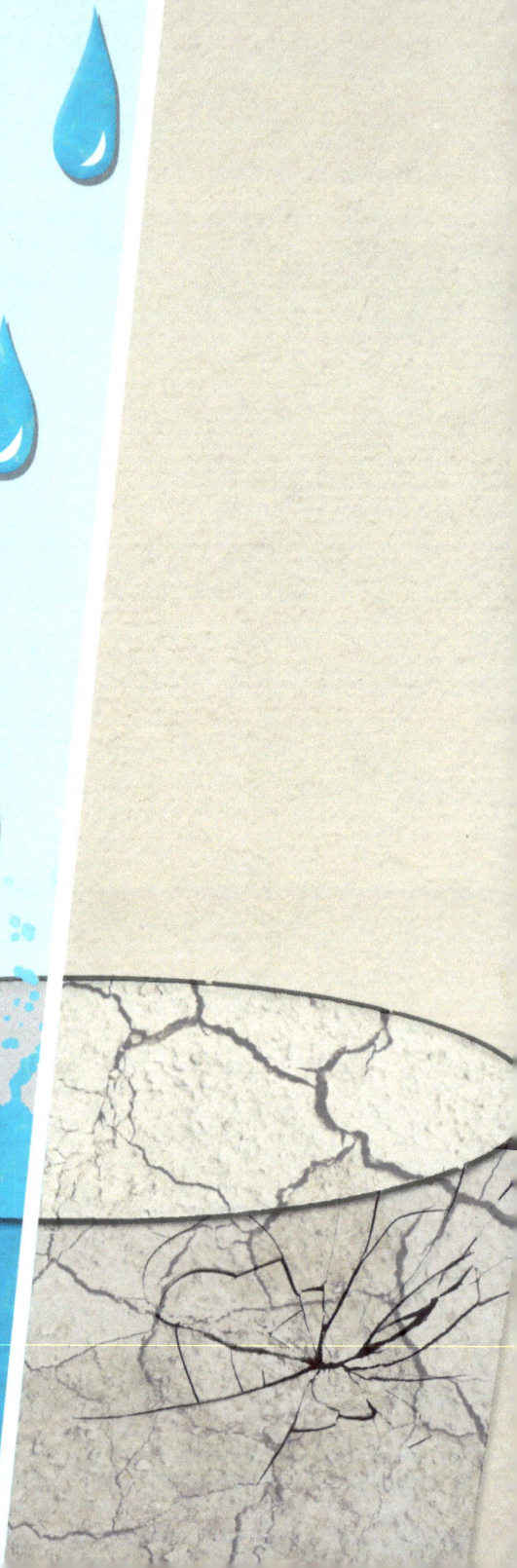

# 3

## The Wonder of Weight Loss

### The Most Overlooked Factor

When I was 28 pounds overweight 10 years ago, I might have been drinking 3 glasses of water in an average day. On top of that, I drank 3 cups of coffee with double cream and sugar just to keep up with my energy demands, even though I had been exercising 3 times a week religiously. One of the big changes I made was to drink about 2.5 L of good quality water every day. With no exception! I am taking my water with me everywhere I go just like I would carry my medication.

Most of us do not look at water being as important as food or exercise. However, we can live for few months without food but will only last about a week without water. Next to the air we breathe, water is the most important element. Every single biochemical process that happens inside our body needs water, period.

........................................

*"Water is the basis of all life. The human body is composed of 25% of solid matter and 75 percent of water. Brain tissue is said to be consist of 85% of water. Even your bones are made of 25% of water."*
*- F. Batmanghelidj, M.D., "Your Body's Many Cries for Water"*
*(www.watercure.com)*

Are you consciously drinking water throughout the day, or allowing yourself go hours without a sip?

Symptoms of moderate to severe dehydration include:

> » Low blood pressure.
> » Fainting.
> » Severe muscle contractions in the arm, legs, stomach, and back.
> » Convulsions.
> » A bloated stomach.
> » Heart failure.
> » Sunken dry eyes, with few or no tears.
> » Skin losing its firmness and becoming wrinkled.
> » A lack of elasticity of the skin (when a pinch of skin stays folded, taking a long time to go back to its normal position).
> » Rapid breathing.
> » Fast, weak pulse.
> » Dark yellow color of urine.
> » Constipation.

### Chronic Dehydration May Be Associated with Weight Gain

### 1. Over eating

According to Dr. F. Batmanghelidj's study and clinical practice on water, the sensation of thirst and hunger are generated simultaneously to indicate the brain's needs. When dehydrated, we do not recognize the sensation of thirst and assume "both indicators" to be the urge to eat. We eat food even when the body should be receiving water. Generally speaking, when you feel hungry and start drinking water first, especially between meals it will help prevent you from over eating and help with weight loss.

Another common phenomenon I have seen is many people who are overweight are drinking a soft drink or fruit juice which contain about 24 - 32g of sugar per glass as well as other chemicals instead of drinking water. By simply switching to water this alone can have the undeniable effect of weight loss.

## 2. Hidden link to high blood sugar

When dehydrated, the blood volume is decreased, which can cause the concentration of your blood sugar level to increase. A high blood sugar level is directly related to other health concerns including weight gain or an inability to lose weight.

## *Other Consequences of Chronic Dehydration*

## 1. Low back pain

I have worked with a lot of clients who have low back pain. A few of them understood that chronic dehydration may have something to do with the pain. In the book *Your Body's Many Cries for Water*, Dr. Batmanghelidj states: "In spinal vertebral joints, including low back, water is not only a lubricant for the contact surfaces, it is held core within the intervertebral space and supports the compression weight of the upper part of body. Once dehydration sets in, all parts of the body begin to suffer. The intervertebral discs and their joints are the first in line."

About 95% of low back pain happens on L5 lumbar disc. The fact is that 75 percent of the weight of the upper body is supported by the water volume that is stored in the 5th disc core. 25 percent is supported by the fibrous materials around the disc. (Dr. F. Batmanghelidj, 1995)

## 2. Potential for hypertension

When the body doesn't get sufficient amounts of water, it compensates by undergoing sodium retention - which is directly related to high blood pressure. If this is not given proper attention, the body then closes some capillary beds which causes increased blood pressure and raises pressure on the arteries.

## 3. Higher toxin levels

Chronic dehydration builds up toxic levels in the body. Cells are more vulnerable to chemical poisoning when in a dehydrated state. One overlooked factor in metabolic syndrome and inflammation is dehydration. (http://drsircus.com/medicine/water/dehydration-3)

Water is a true miracle and the least expensive drug you can have to lose weight and improve your physical and mental health.

## *Drinking Tips:*

1.  Water quality is important. Tap water is not the best choice for a number of reasons.

    According to Sherry A. Rogers, M.D.'s study, tap water:

    » contains **fluoride**. It is known to cause excessive calcification not only in arteries but joints and ligaments, and contributes to many forms of cancer and osteoporosis.
    » contains **chlorine**. Chlorine is a free radical initiator that elevates cholesterol and causes accelerated aging. Statistical analysis and comprehensive articles have documented how the chlorine in your water promotes not only arteriosclerosis (hardening of the arteries), but various types of cancers of the rectum and bladder.
    » contains **industrial chemicals, drug residuals** and **heavy metals** from pipes.

2.  I follow Dr. F. Batmanghelidj's advice. We should drink half of our body weight (lb.) in ounces. If you weigh 150 lbs., you may need to drink 75 ounces every day.

3.  Figure out how many cups you drink on an average day. Start drinking 1 - 2 extra cups on top of what you drink now for 3 weeks to avoid going to the washroom too often. After 3 weeks, up it another 1 - 2 cups for 3 weeks consistently.

4. The key is consistency. Find a way that works for you so you can make it habit. For instance, I have a client who makes 6 marks on a 1.5 L bottle while at work. By the end of the day, she has to finish the whole bottle before going home.

5. Drink 1 - 2 cups of room temperature or warm water first thing in the morning every day. Once I started that, years ago, it helped me get rid of my morning urge for coffee. Most of my friends and clients feel the same after simply drinking water first thing in the morning.

6. Drink a cup of water 15 minutes before a meal to assist in digestion. Do not drink water while eating as water can dilute the stomach acid and weaken the digestion. After a meal, wait for about 45 minutes, then drink one cup every hour.

7. Your skin is the largest organ. If you shower with chlorine and fluoride contained tap water, you are drinking it too. It is a good idea to find a shower filter that can filter out chlorine and other residues.

---

### ·Take Action·

*Intentional thought: "I always remember to drink the right amount of water every day."*

1. Drink 1 - 2 cups of room temperature water every morning.

2. Take your body weight in pounds and divide by 2. That is how much water in ounces you need every day.

3. Figure out how much water you drink in an average day, start to drink 1-2 cups more every day for 2 weeks and then add another 1-2 cups until you reach your ideal intake. Make it a habit.

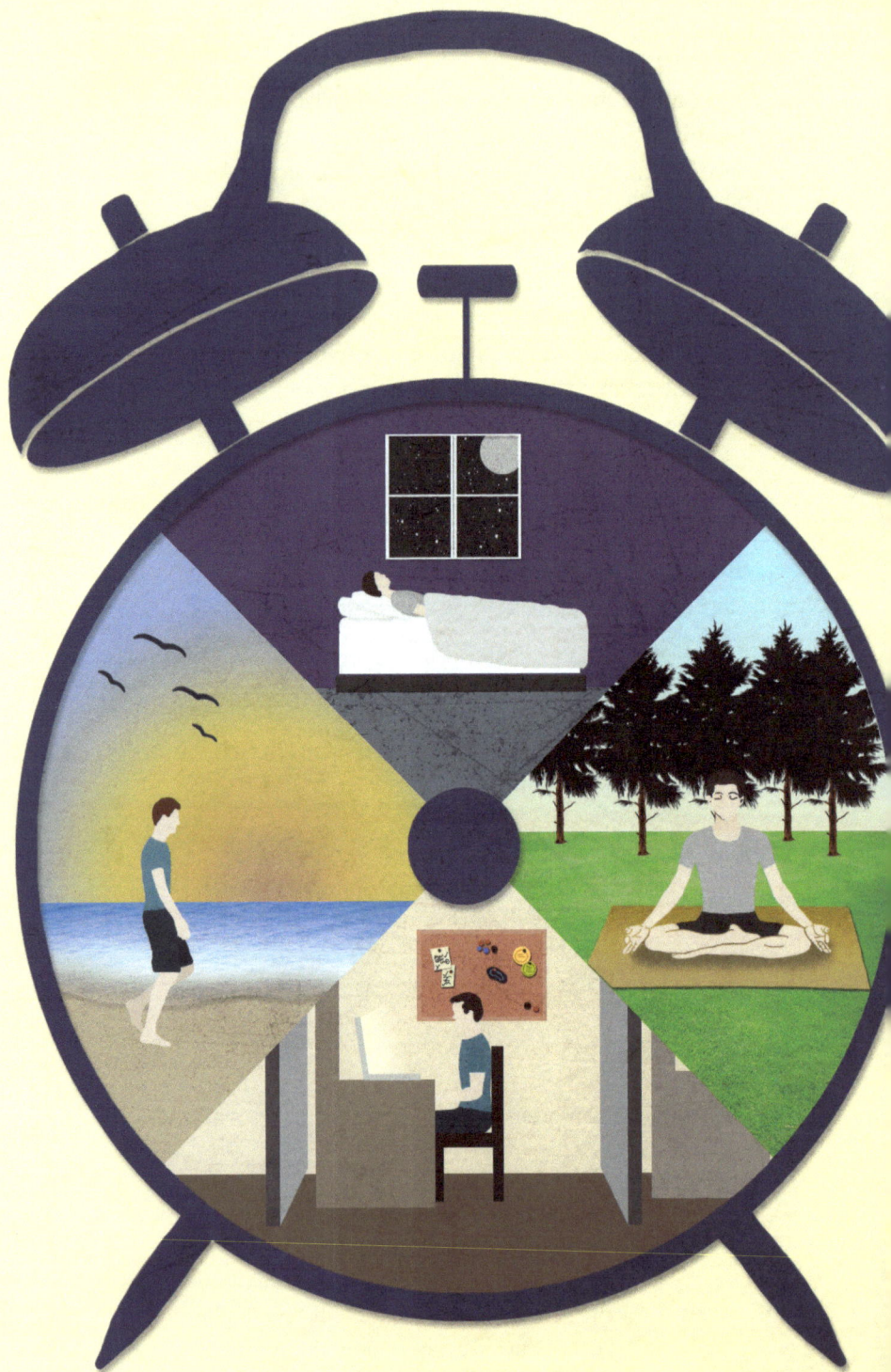

# 4

## *Transform Your Body Effortlessly with Sleep*

### *The Shocking Facts*

For a very long time before I was 40, I always went to bed after midnight. It was okay for quite a while. Then I started to find it more difficult to get up in the morning. I was on 3 coffees every day to keep me going. One of the biggest parts of the transformation of my body and life was rebuilding my sleep/wake cycle after 40.

Now when I work with my clients over 40, I find 90% of them are not having enough sleep, or not going to bed at the proper time. The first step I recommend is to work on sleep habits while starting an exercise program.

Based on US National Sleep Foundation, National Department of Transportation, and Centers of Disease Control and Prevention:

» 40 million people have a chronic sleep disorder.
» $18 billion is the cost to employer in lost productivity due to sleep loss.
» 62% of American adults experience a sleep problem a few nights per week.
» 70 million adults suffer from insomnia.

Interestingly enough, there are 70 million people, two-thirds of population in the U.S., who suffer from insomnia, and also two-thirds of the population is overweight. Personally I believe sleep loss is the root cause of being overweight, having a blood sugar problem, hormone imbalance, chronic pain and inflammation, and even cancer.

As much as I like discussing exercise programs at the beginning of this book, I strongly believe without assessing and resetting the sleep/wake cycle, it is almost impossible to see a good result from exercising alone. The longer you have the wrong sleep/wake cycle, the more it may damage your body, and the more urgent it becomes to correct it.

## *Understanding the Body's Internal Clock*

According to Wikipedia, "Sleep is a heightened anabolic state, accentuating the growth and rejuvenation of the immune, nervous, skeletal and muscular systems. It is observed in all mammals, all birds, and many reptiles, amphibians, and fish."

Our internal 24-hour sleep/wake cycle, otherwise known as your biological clock or circadian rhythm, is processed in the area of the brain known as the suprachiasmatic nucleus (SCN), in response to light and dark. For example, at night as SCN receives the information from the optic nerve of less light, it triggers the brain to produce more melatonin so you can sleep. This is why you should not watch TV or use a computer before trying to go to sleep as they are too bright and too stimulating.

......................................................

*"The hormones melatonin and prolactin are major players in your mind-body-planet connection. They communicate with your immune system and metabolic energy system about light-dark cycles. Insulin and prolactin orchestrate the brain chemistry governing serotonin and dopamine in your brain, to control your behavior and mood. Seratonin and dopamine control your behavior regarding food and sex. Bottom line: Not enough sleep makes you fat, hungry, impotent, hypertensive, and cancerous, with a bad heart".*
*- T.S. Wiley, author of "Lights Out, Sleep, Sugar and Survival"*

## *Chronic Sleep Lost Leads to*

» Fatigue, lethargy, lack of motivation even depression - Moodiness and irritability.
» Inability to cope with stress.
» Compromised immunity; frequent colds and infections.
» Weight grain.
» Concentration and memory problems.
» Difficulty making decisions.
» Very suppressed appetite in the morning.
» Increased risk of diabetes, heart disease, and other health problems, even cancer.

## *Myth and Truth about Sleep*

### Myth 1: I can make up the sleep lost by sleeping more during the weekend

Although this sleeping pattern will help relieve part of the sleep debt, it will not completely make up for the lack of sleep. Furthermore, sleeping later on the weekends can affect your sleep/wake cycle so that it is much harder to go to sleep at the right time on Sunday nights and get up early on Monday mornings. How many of us experience "Black Mondays"?

### Myth 2: As long as I get 8 hours sleep, it doesn't matter when I go to bed

This is very common belief. However it is not the way the body works. We are a part of nature. All body functions follow nature: seasons, dark and light. Ignoring it can bring unwanted dis-ease.

## Myth 3: Just sleeping one hour less doesn't affect my day-time functioning

You may not be noticeably sleepy during the day, but losing even one hour of sleep can affect your ability to think properly and respond quickly, especially if you're doing it on a daily basis. It also compromises your cardiovascular health, energy balance, and ability to fight infections.

### *Sleep with a 24 Hour Cycle*

In Chinese medicine, which has information based on observing the interaction between the human body and nature over thousands of years, the 12 major meridian systems (Lung meridians, Large Intestine meridians, Spleen meridians, Stomach meridians, Heart meridians, Small Intestine meridians, Kidney meridians, Urinary Bladder meridians, Pericardium meridians, Triple Burner meridians, Liver meridians and Gall Bladder meridians) are all working with a 24 hour cycle. Every two hours one of these meridian systems is at its peak.

At night for example, from 11:00 PM–1:00 AM the Gall Bladder meridian system is at its peak; 1:00 AM–3:00 AM the Liver meridian system is at its peak. If you always wake up between 1:00 AM and 3:00 AM, it may indicate that you have impaired liver function. 3:00 AM–5:00 AM the Lung meridian system is working at its best. And the Large Intestine meridian system is very active between 5:00 AM–7:00 AM. That is why having 1-2 cups of water first thing in the morning will help with a bowl movement.

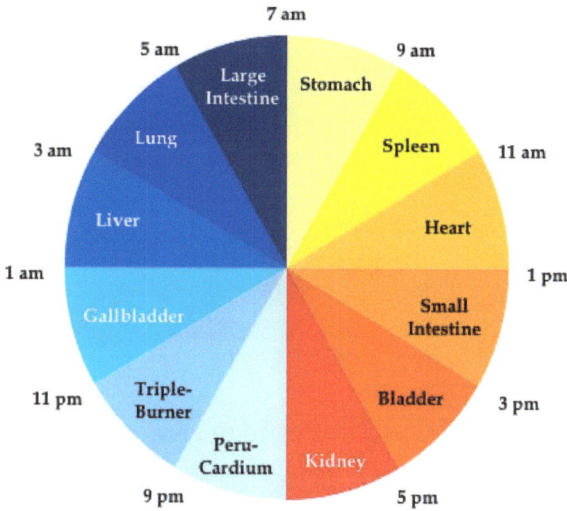

(http://freakgirl.com/blog/wp-content/uploads/2011/07/chinese_body_clock.png)

## *Sleep with the Seasons*

Written over 2000 years ago in China, *Yellow Emperors Classic Medicine*, discovered sleeping with the seasons and with a 24 hour cycle is the best way to attain optimal health and to prevent disease.

**Spring:** go to sleep early and get up early. (ie. 10:30 PM - 6:30 AM)

**Summer:** go to sleep late and get up early. (ie. 11:00 PM – 6:00 AM)

**Fall:** go to sleep early and get up early. (ie. 10:30 PM - 6:30 AM)

**Winter:** go to sleep early and get up late. (ie. 10:00 PM – 7:00 AM)

This all makes perfect sense to me as our sleep and wake-up hormones are in tune with the Sun and the Moon.

I personally go to sleep quite early in winter, like 9:30 PM or at the latest by 10:00 PM. It is the key to maintaining my body weight in winter, as artificial light to the body means summer and carbohydrates. The later I stay up under artificial light, the more I want to eat. Once spring hits, I slowly adapt my bed-time to 10:15 PM then 10:30 PM until we reach summer. I even go to bed by 11:00 PM in the middle of summer for a month. Then when it becomes dark earlier as it approaches fall I resume going to bed by 10:30 PM, then 10:00 PM and 9:30 PM. I have been doing this for a few years now. My body weight stays stable throughout the entire year. Moreover, I never catch any seasonal flu at all.

### Tips On Restoring Sleep/Wake Cycle

1. Adapt your bed-time according to the seasons.

2. When you decide to change, start with a 15 minute increment at a time. Do it for 3 weeks, and then another 15 minute increment for 3 weeks. This way, the body adapts slowly and effortlessly.

3. Stop watching TV, using the computer and other electronic devices at least 30 minutes before bed-time. Research shows 90% of people who have insomnia either watch TV or use electronic items 60 minutes before going to bed.

4. Avoid coffee after lunch. Also avoid sugary foods and alcohol at night as they are powerful stimulants.

5. Eat balanced protein and vegetables at dinner. Too much starchy food can cause low blood sugar at night and keep you awake. If you feel hungry before bed, try to have a little bit of a protein rich food, such as almond butter.

6. Sleep in a dark room which has no TV or other electronic devices.

7. Do not over-exercise at night, especially when it is already dark. Stretches however would be beneficial to a good night's sleep. Or do less than 30 minutes of short circuit training.

·········································Take Action··········································

*Intentional thought: "My body works at its best when I go to sleep by 10:30PM."*

1. Minimize using electronic devices such as TV, cell phone and computer in your bedroom.

2. Stop watching TV or working on your computer at least 30 minutes before bed-time.

3. If you commit to going to bed early, start with 15 - 30 minute increments at a time. For example, go to bed at 11:45 PM then 11:30 PM if you normally go to bed at 12:00 AM. Follow the same schedule for 3 weeks. Then another 15 to 30 minutes earlier for another 3 weeks. It takes about 9 to 12 weeks to be at 10:30 PM.

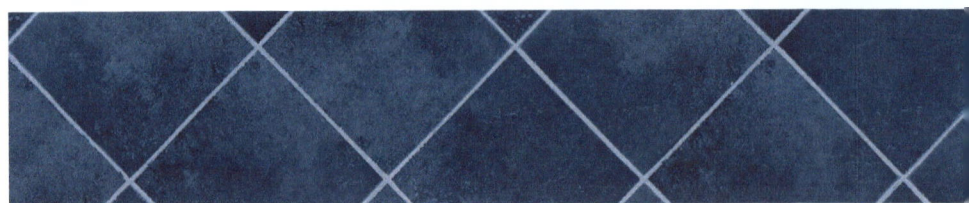

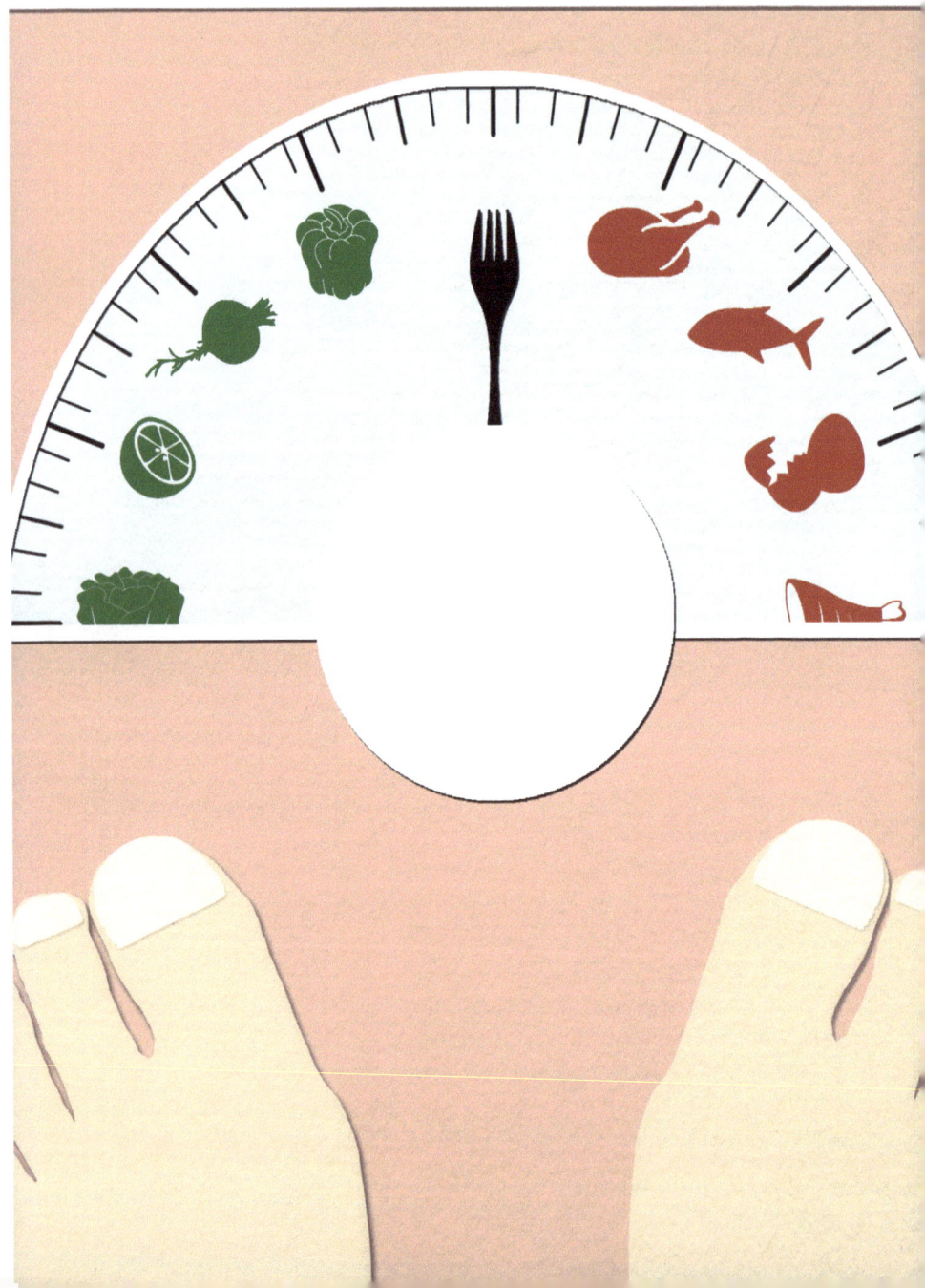

# 5

## 7 Simple Ways of Eating Right for YOU

*"Let food be thy medicine and medicine be thy food."*
*- Hippocrates, 460 - 377 BC*

.................................................

Believe or not, food is essential for health and performance. It not only provides energy for daily physical demands, but also it is used by the body to produce hormones and neurotransmitters for mental and emotional balance.

Once I decided to change my diet 10 years ago, I followed official food guidelines for two years. The typical day was cereal or oatmeal with low fat milk in the morning, a big salad with some chicken or a whole wheat wrap for lunch, and rice with stir-fry vegetables and chicken or beef for dinner. It sounds healthy right? However I was tired and sleepy after eating; I was hungry almost every hour if I didn't have a snack; I was craving salty foods like chips, as well as wine at night; my skin was very dry; my hair was falling out easily. Most of all I was moody. I might have been unknowingly hypoglycemic.

It led me to spend the last 8 years studying and practicing nutrition to figure out what works for me, as an individual. I am not a dietitian, I cannot tell you what to eat. However I do believe that no diet/nutrition expert or health professional can replace my body's innate intelligence. I don't care what the diet trend is out there, for me, the diet is not right if one is feeling hungry one hour after eating, feeling tired and moody, or craving more food.

Now I eat almost the opposite of what I was eating. In a typical day I eat organic pork sausage or chicken wings with celery and carrots in the morning; same food for lunch, and at dinner it would be fish with spinach. I feel full and satisfied after each meal for as long as 3 - 4 hours, and I'm energetic all day long.

I strongly believe that we are all different in terms of our genetic traits, such as appearance, height, and metabolic rate. On top of that we have different mental and physical needs. We are not supposed to eat the same. Unfortunately we did not enter this world with an owner's manual. So you are the only one who is able to judge if your diet is right for you, as your body is communicating with you all the time. In this chapter, I will share with you the four big myths which were road blocks for me and 7 simple steps that helped me with my own diet, so you can work on yours.

### Four Big Myths about Diet

### 1. Calorie Counting Myth

As reported by www.mercola.com, David Kirchoff, president of Weight Watchers, the world's largest diet company, recently said on their website: "Calorie counting has become unhelpful. When we have a 100-calorie apple in one hand and a 100-calorie pack of cookies in the other, and we view them as being 'the same' because the calories are the same, it says everything that needs to be said about the limitations of just using calories in guiding food choices."

The calorie counting myth has helped the food processing industry and weight-loss industry make billions of dollars in recent decades. Are obesity, heart disease, diabetes, and cancer getting better or worse? Go figure! Now it is time to rethink it.

It is far more important to look at the source of calories as opposed to counting them. In my research and self-experimentation in the past 8 years, eating high quality and nutrient dense food with the right ratio of starch, protein and fat for my body is the key to maintaining blood sugar balance, hormonal balance and energy balance which result in my healthy weight.

I stopped counting calories 8 years ago. I only look at the food source, quality and ratio of starch, protein and fat when it comes to choosing what I eat. Not only have I lost 28 lbs. but I am relaxed and enjoying what I eat.

## 2. Saturated Fat and Cholesterol Myth

I was scared to death when eating saturated fat and cholesterol 10 years ago, believing it would make me fat and unhealthy. However when I was eating a diet of low fat and cholesterol for two years, I was hungry all the time; I was moody; my skin was dry and my sex drive was low. Then I started question about my diet. In 2005, I was introduced to a systematic approach called *Metabolic Typing Diet* by William Wolcott. I figured out I was a protein type which means my body was sensitive to starchy food. I had to eat more fat and protein to slow down the blood sugar conversion; I started slowly adding more high quality fat and protein to my diet. I actually felt better and better. I became leaner, energetic and less hungry.

For the past several decades, the low fat / low cholesterol trend has been appearing in front of my eyes. Obesity, heart disease, diabetes, and the rate of cancer have been surprisingly increasing, not decreasing. The fact is, from 1910 to 1970, the proportion of traditional animal fat in the American diet declined from 83% to 62%, and butter consumption plummeted from 18 pounds per person per year to 4 pounds. While the percentage of dietary vegetable oils in the form of margarine, shortening and refined oils increased about 400%. At the same time the consumption of sugar and processed food increased about 60%. It is obvious to me that it is not the saturated fat which is responsible for the increasing number of people with obesity, heart disease and cancer, rather it is refined vegetable oils, processed food and sugar.

Low fat diets push high sugar / high starch consumption, which lead to a blood sugar imbalance for most people, and further results in an energy imbalance and weight gain. Eating fat and protein rich food gives the body satiety as it is digested slowly. "As a result of the presence of fat in the small intestine, special hormones are produced that prevent the hunger contractions" (Mary G. Enig, Ph.D., *Know Your Fats*). I am one of those people who is sensitive to starchy food and need an ample amount of fat and protein in any given meal.

Low fat diets may result in fat soluble vitamins like A, D, E, and K deficiency.

Cholesterol is a vital substance for physical and mental health. According to Uffe Ravnskov, MD, PhD.

> » Cholesterol in cell membranes makes cells waterproof so there can be different chemistry on the inside and outside of the cell.
> » The body produces three to four times more cholesterol than you eat. The production of cholesterol increases when you eat a little cholesterol and decreases when you eat a lot.
> » Cholesterol protects us against depression; it plays a role in the utilization of serotonin, the body's "feel good" hormone.
> » Cholesterol is the precursor of vitamin D, which is formed by the action of UV-B light on cholesterol in the skin.
> » Cholesterol is needed in the creation of all sex hormones, such as testosterone, estrogen and progesterone, and many other hormones.
> » Cholesterol is nature's repair substance, used to repair wounds, including tears and irritations in the arteries.
> (www.westonaprice.org)

I have been eating high quality protein and fat with a small amount of vegetables or rice for 8 years now and I haven't gotten fatter but rather leaner. I can feel the energy flow increasing smoothly after eating instead of feeling a sugar rush which then makes me sleepy and tired.

## 3. One Fits All Approach

*"One man's food is another's poison."*
*- Lucretious, 99 - 55 B.C.*

.................................................

One of the biggest mistakes is to follow a diet that works for another and to believe it will work for you the same way. I am sure any diet out there, whether it is low fat diet, Atkins diet, South Beach diet, or vegetarian diet, only works for certain individuals, but not for all. We are all different in terms of color, height, appearances, size, metabolic rate, and mental / physical demands. Even our cultural and geographic backgrounds are different. We are not meant to eat the same. In *Biochemical Individuality*, published in 1956, Dr. Roger, J. Williams discovered scientific evidence of human differences in anatomical variations, blood composition, enzyme patterns, and endocrine activities. He suggested "self-selection of food" as a means of satisfying individual nutrition needs, and connecting with the body's wisdom. I often get asked "what should I eat". Unfortunately I cannot tell you what to eat, but I can give you basic principles that have helped me, so you can find the answer for yourself.

## 4. Whole Wheat is Healthy

I ate whole wheat cereals and whole wheat bread or whole wheat pasta every day 10 years ago believing it was healthy. But I was bloated and gassy quite often. I was hungry all the time. On top of that, I had chronic knee pain when I stepped up and down stairs, and skin rashes on my hands.

Whole wheat products are consumed about 133 pounds per person per year in the USA. It is such a common belief that eating whole wheat cereal, bread, and pasta is a healthy choice. However, Dr. William Davis, a cardiologist, wrote a book called *Wheat Belly - Lose the Wheat, Lose the Weight, and Find Your Path Back to Health* in 2011.

Dr. Davis provided clinical studies and the extraordinary results after putting thousands of his patients on wheat-free diet regimens, which led him to believe that wheat is the root cause of obesity, diabetes, heart disease and many auto-immune conditions. In 2013 another book *Grain Brain: The Surprising Truth about Wheat, Carbs and Sugar - Your Brain's Silent Killers* by Dr. David Perlmutter, Neurologist and Fellow of American College of Nutrition, pointed out that a whole wheat, high carb, and high sugar diet may contribute to Alzheimer's and other neurological conditions, such as depression, brain fog. To summarize their research and clinical findings:

» Wheat is an appetite stimulant: it makes you want more - more bagels, muffins, tacos, sandwiches, pizza etc. It makes you want both wheat-containing and non-wheat-containing foods. And on top of that, for some people wheat is a drug, or at least yields peculiar drug-like neurological effects. People on a diet of wheat on average consume extra 400 calories than those who are off wheat. The average person loses 26 lbs. on the Wheat Belly Diet within 6 months.

» Wheat disturbs the blood sugar balance. In fact, just two slices of whole wheat bread increases blood sugar to a level higher than eating a candy bar. A high blood sugar level provokes visceral fat accumulation.

» Wheat causes inflammation in the body, from gut to brain, joints to muscles, and over the course of years develops auto-immune conditions. Autoimmunity is becoming the number three cause of morbidity and mortality.

» It is estimated up to 50% of the population has non-celiac gluten sensitivity (www.doctoroz.com). Symptoms can be categorized as: Digestive symptoms:
  » Frequent bloating or gas.
  » Diagnosed with IBS or acid reflux.
  » Daily diarrhea or chronic constipation.

Neurological & Skeletal Symptoms:
- » Migraine or headaches.
- » Joint pain or aches.
- » Brain fog.

Hormonal & Immune Symptoms:
- » Depression or anxiety.
- » Ongoing fatigue.
- » Chronic eczema or acne.

At the first world online Gluten Summit in November 2013 organized by Dr. Thomas O'Bryan (www.theglutensummit.com), Dr. Alessio Fasano, the leading MD from the Center for Celiac Research and Treatment made a strong statement: **"Gluten is not digestible by any human"**.

## 7 Simple Steps to Eat Right for YOU

**1. Eliminate processed foods. Get local organic vegetables, fruits and meats.**

When it comes to choosing foods, it is very simple: more nutrients and fewer toxins. In eating the food that grows, you will grow. Eat high quality wholesome food in its original state. Organic is the best choice.

Don'ts:

- » Sugar, high-fructose corn syrup and artificial sweeteners which can be found in soft drinks, fruit drinks and most low fat products
- » Margarine and vegetable oils.
- » Processed wheat products: cereals, muffins, cookies, bread and pasta.

» GMO (Genetically Modified Organism) food and ingredients: corn, soy, canola are the big threes.
» Avoid foods with a long list of ingredient that you cannot pronounce.
» Boxed, frozen dinners.

Dos:

» Unprocessed honey, maple syrup, or stevia to replace sugar.
» Organic butter, extra virgin olive oil, cold pressed sesame oil, coconut oil, gees.
» Local (organic whenever possible) fruits and vegetable.
» Free run (organic) eggs.
» Grass fed beef.
» Organic free range chicken.
» Wild fish.

## 2. Be the authority on your own diet

**Four Signs of Eating Right or Wrong:** There is too much information about diet out there that is confusing. It doesn't matter what diet you are on, it has to provide the body with the right amount of protein, starch and fat for sustained energy, a stable blood sugar level and balanced hormones. I always use these four signs to guide me on a meal-to-meal basis.

Within one to two hours after a meal, simply ask yourself:

| Signs | Right | Wrong |
|---|---|---|
| Am I Full or Satisfied? Do I Have Sweet Cravings? | » Feel full and satisfied<br>» Stop eating, don't want more<br>» Do not have sweet cravings | » Feel physically full, but still hungry<br>» Don't feel satisfied; feel something is still missing<br>» Have a desire for sweets |
| Am I Hungry? Do I Need a Snack? | » Do not get hungry soon after eating<br>» Do not need a snack before the next meal | » Feel hungry again soon after eating<br>» Need a snack between meals |
| How is My Energy Level? | » Energy is restored after eating<br>» Have good and sustained energy and a sense of well-being | » Energy drop, fatigue, exhaustion, sleepiness or drowsiness<br>» Feel hyper, but exhausted "underneath"<br>» Become hyper, jittery, shaky, or nervous |
| What is My Mental/ Emotional State? | » Sense of feeling refueled and restored<br>» Uplifted emotionally<br>» Improved clarity and acuity of mind<br>» Normalization of thought processes | » Mentally slow, sluggish, spacy<br>» Inability to think quickly or clearly<br>» Hyper, overly rapid thoughts<br>» Hypo state: apathy, depression, or sadness<br>» Hyper state: anxiety, obsessiveness, fearfulness, anger, short tempered, or irritable |

(Adapted from The Metabolic Typing Diet, page 265, William Wolcott and Trish Fahey, 2000)

**Understand Your Metabolic Type:** When I read William Wolcott and Trish Fahey's book *The Metabolic Typing Diet* eight years ago, I knew I found the answer for my two year struggle with my diet. "Metabolic Type is specific, individualized, genetic-based patterns of biochemical individuality that defines one's metabolic 'designed limits' and dictates an individual response to, and requirements for nutritional substances." (www.healthexcel.com) It explains why I see people lose weight and do really well with a low fat diet, where others achieve the same results by being on a high fat, high protein diet. Understanding your Metabolic Type is like knowing what kind of engine your car is equipped with. If you have a diesel engine, you would need diesel gas in order to perform at optimal levels; Eating according to your Metabolic Type is like putting the right gas in your body to fuel your unique engine. I have been following this system for the past 8 years. Not only have I lost all the unnecessary weight totaling 28 lbs., but I have also gained a great deal of energy and mental focus that sustains me all day long, without any craving for sweets, chips or red wine. A quick overview of the different Metabolic Types is listed below:

| Metabolic Type | Diet | Macro-nutrient ratio |
|---|---|---|
| Protein Type | » High in protein<br>» Heavy, fatty, high purine proteins, such as beef (and liver), bacon and chicken legs<br>» High fats and oils like butter and nuts<br>» Non starchy vegetables like spinach, celery and mushrooms | » 70% proteins and fats<br>» 30% carbohydrates |
| Carb Type | » Low in protein<br>» Light, lean, low purine proteins, such as chicken breast, turkey breast and cod<br>» Low fats and oils<br>» Medium starchy carbohydrates like zucchini, brussel sprouts and leafy greens | » 40% proteins and fats<br>» 60% carbohydrates |
| Mixed Type | » Mixture of high-fat, high-protein and low-fat, low-protein<br>» Requires relatively equal ratios of proteins, fat and carbohydrates | » 50% proteins and fats<br>» 50% carbohydrates |

(Adapted from The Metabolic Typing Diet, William Wolcott and Trish Fahey, 2000)

**How to Find Your Metabolic Type:** Through Metabolic Typing, a systematic methodology developed by William Wocott, you can find out your unique Metabolic Type and the optimal way to eat for you as an individual. There are three ways: One, complete the questionnaires included in the book *The Metabolic Typing Diet* by William Wolcott and Trish Fasey and follow its guidance; Two, take an online questionnaire or find a certified Metabolic Typing Advisor at www.healthexcel.com; Three, simply download my free personal report "Metabolic Typing: the Key to My Diet" at www.wisdomfitbyoprae.com.

**Optimize Your Macronutrient Ratio:** Typically, finding your optimal diet involves shifting the ratio of protein, fat and carbohydrate. One diet doesn't fit all. Please note that even if you and I are both protein types, it doesn't mean we have to eat the same ratio of fat, protein vs. carbohydrates. Only use the ratio in the table as your starting point. Use four signs of eating right or wrong to figure out the best ratio for your body within your metabolic type. Your body is dynamic, meaning that when your physical demands change or the season changes, your macronutrient requirements change too. For example, after an intensive workout, I usually add one extra serving of carbohydrate. In summer, I eat a mixed type of an almost one-to-one ratio of protein, fat and carbohydrates, and I eat more lean meat and fish. While in winter, I eat more fat and protein and fewer starchy vegetables. Just listen to your body, it doesn't lie!

### 3. Avoid GMO foods and ingredients

GMO (Genetically Modified Organism) is the result of a laboratory process of taking genes from one species and inserting them into another in an attempt to obtain a desired trait or characteristic. For example, a GMO crop contains genes from a certain herbicide so it can resist the same herbicide while it is sprayed. I personally would avoid food contaminated with any GMO ingredients.

» There are many countries banning GMOs, such as Japan, New Zealand, Germany, Ireland, France, Switzerland, and more.

» Reported on www.responsibletechnology.org, In 2009, AAEM (the American Academy of Environmental Medicine) stated that, "Several animal studies indicate serious health risks associated with genetically modified (GM) food, including infertility, immune problems, accelerated aging, faulty insulin regulation, and changes in major organs and the gastrointestinal system." The AAEM has asked physicians to advise all patients to avoid GM food.

» Currently major GMO crops in the USA include soy (94%), cotton (90%), canola (90%), sugar beets (95%), and corn (88%). Nearly all Canadian canola is GM, as is a large portion of the country's soy and corn.

» Other sources of GMOs: meat, eggs and dairy products from animals that feed on GMO crops, dairy products from cows injected with rbGH (a GM hormone, not approved in Canada), soy protein, soy lecithin, corn starch, corn syrup and high fructose corn syrup.

» You can download a non GMO shopping guide at www.responsibletechnology.org.

## 4. Take time to chew your food

Have you thought that even though you eat the best source of meats, fish and vegetables, it doesn't mean anything to your body until the food is broken down into molecules like amino acids (a breakdown from meats), fatty acids (a breakdown from fats) and glucose (a breakdown from starchy foods), fructose (a breakdown from fruits) and lactose (a breakdown from diary). Maintaining good digestion on a meal-to-meal basis is as important as what you eat. You are not just what you eat, you are also what you digest.

Digestion is a part of a parasympathetic process meaning a calm and relaxed environment helps the body do the job more effectively. Chewing food properly not only helps breakdown the food to smaller particles that can be exposed to saliva, allowing the body to absorb more nutrients, but also the body has the time to signal to you when you are full. It is a perfect way to manage your weight. Thin people usually eat slowly. Here are some tips:

» Find a quiet place, away from the computer and desk.
» Take 10 deep breaths.
» Chew your food until it is liquefied.
» Don't add more food until you finish the current bite.
» Bless your food, taste and feel it.
» Take another 10 deep breaths when you finish eating.

## 5. Always eat with the seasons

Our ancestors have been eating with the seasons for generation after generation. Chinese ancestors and healing masters believe that seasonal food has cooling, warming or heating properties that help our body cooperate with the weather and achieve optimal health.

In spring, focus on tender, leafy vegetables such as spinach, kale, asparagus and dandelion greens. In summer, fill your diet with light, cooling vegetables and fruits such as berries, summer squash, cucumber, tomatoes, peppermint and cilantro. Fish and sea food are also perfect for summer. Fall brings the autumn harvest and warming foods such as sweet potatoes, onions, carrots, and ginger. Winter calls for food that has warm properties, such root vegetables, as well as animal foods such as chicken, beef and lamb.

## 6. Rotate your food

It is common to see people eating the same food every morning, every lunch and dinner. It is boring and limiting. By rotating your food, you not only get more variety of food but also prevent the body from developing food allergies. For example, I have seen many of my clients getting so much better in terms of energy and chronic inflammation after limiting the amount of cheese they eat every day. Be aware that you may become allergic to what you are addicted to.

I always change up my protein source and vegetables throughout the week. For example, I eat chicken and green beans on Monday, lamb and sweat potatoes on Tuesday, beef and cauliflower on Wednesday, and fish and asparagus on Thursday. Then I rotate them again or try something different. I also don't have dairy every day. I have raw organic cheese twice a week and goat's milk a couple of times a week. Milk and cheese are on the top three lists for allergies. Remember if you love a certain kind of food, rotate it.

## 7. 80/20 rule

If you follow the right choices 80% of the time, your body can deal with the bad choices you make 20% of the time.

Having said that, one day a week you can enjoy a "cheat day". My cheat foods would be organic dark chocolate or home-made organic pop-corn with organic butter. Nobody is perfect. We all have our moments.

### *Other Cautions*

### Coffee

I enjoy high quality organic espresso or coffee as much as any coffee lover, just like you. Coffee does aid one's workout and mental performance, like writing. It also contains beneficial antioxidants. However, over-doing it could have negative effects, such as over-stimulating the sympathetic nervous system which can lead to adrenal fatigue. Coffee is also a powerful stimulant that is very addictive. According to Paul Chek, Holistic Health Practitioner, coffee is very stressful to the female physiology! It is disruptive to females with any form of menstrual irregularity and particularly troublesome for premenopausal, menopausal, and postmenopausal women.

So find your threshold for coffee. I usually have a single shot of espresso (organic, if possible) per day, occasionally two. I can still have a good night's sleep and feel calm during the day.

## Alcohol

Most physicians tell their patients that having a few glasses of wine per day is okay. However I personally disagree for the following reasons:

» Alcohol stresses the body more than you think, as it is absorbed directly and quickly into the stomach and small intestines causing not only damage to the gut lining, but also a spike in blood sugar, releasing insulin, which leads to hypoglycemia (low blood sugar). When your body is under a hypoglycemic state, it relies on the stress hormone cortisol to deal with it. That's why you may wake up in the middle of the night. Moreover, too much cortisol leads to weight gain.
» It disturbs your liver function. Additional enzymes have to be released to metabolize alcohol.
» It dehydrates the body. Some people have headaches in the morning after drinking the night before.
» When consumed in the evening, it may reduce the natural release of growth hormone. Research has shown that as little as one glass of alcohol can reduce the production of growth hormone by 63%.

My take on alcohol:

» No more than 2 glasses of 6 ounces per week.
» Never drink alcohol on an empty stomach. Have some high quality organic fat and protein ahead of time.
» Consider alcohol as a super carb. When drinking, choose a meal with more protein, healthy fat and fewer carbs.

## Salt free

We all know that the excessive intake of salt can cause health problems, but too little can be detrimental as well. It is very common in my observation that quite a number of people over 40 are on a salt limited diet. However an adequate amount of unrefined sea salt, like Celtic Sea Salt, or Himalayan Salt is essential to health and fitness.

» Natural salt is vital to the extraction of excess acidity from the cells of body, particularly brain cells.
» Natural salt is needed for making stomach acids (hydrochloric acid) to help with digestion. A salt-restricted diet can cause you to end up with hypochlorhydria (low hydrochloric acid), and compromised digestion.
» Natural salt can aid in the prevention of muscle cramps.
» Natural salt clears the lungs of mucus plugs and sticky phlegm, particularly in those suffering from asthma. (Paul Chek, *How to Eat, Move and Be Healthy*, page 77)

In Chinese medicine, adequate salt supports the adrenal glands and kidneys. I have a client who was on a no salt diet for 3 years and developed adrenal exhaustion. She was experiencing extreme low energy in the afternoons. Since she started adding a pinch of unprocessed sea salt to her water in the afternoon, she has felt so much better.

I always use high quality unprocessed sea salt for cooking. I carry salt with me and use just a pinch in my water after a sweat-producing workout. It is my cost-effective sports drink.

**Microwave**

I stopped using a microwave 8 years ago after my own research. I try not to stay in the room when someone is using a microwave to heat food. You can find a complete report "The Proven Danger of Microwave Ovens" at http://www.globalhealingcenter.com/health-hazards-to-know-about/microwave-ovens-the-proven-dangers.
This information may convince you to throw out your microwave oven, as it did to me:

» Continually eating food heated in a microwave oven causes long term permanent brain damage by "shorting out" electrical impulses in the brain.
» The human body cannot metabolize or break down the unknown byproducts created by microwaved food.

» Continual ingestion of microwaved food causes immune system deficiencies through lymph gland and blood serum alterations.
» Minerals, vitamins, and nutrients in microwaved food are reduced or altered so that the human body gets little or no benefit.
» The prolonged eating of microwaved food causes cancerous cells to increase in human blood.

I use a traditional oven and toaster-oven at home. If there is no toaster-oven at the place where I bring my own food, I just eat it at room temperature and chew slowly so it can be warmed up in my mouth.

·····Take Action·····

*Intentional thought: "It is easy to make a change in my diet. It is done."*

1. Spend one hour each week watching video lectures or reading one of the books listed in page 126 (References and Resources).

2. Work on one thing at a time and take a small step every day. For example, when I decided to cut out bread, I started to only consume one slice of bread a day, which is half of what I normally would eat, for about 3 weeks. Then I had one slice every other day for 3 weeks, a few times a week, once a week, once every two weeks, once a month. This is what I recommend you do as the less you eat, the less you crave.

3. Write a food journal and start connecting your instincts. Make a check mark on the foods that help you feel great and that last more than 3 hours. Soon you will have a list of meals that work best for you.

.

# *Part II*

# Building True Fitness After 40

*"Life is movement." "Stop moving and we start dying."*
*- Paul Chek, author of*
*How to Eat, Move and Be Healthy*

..............................................

*By now I am sure you have tons of energy by thinking right, breathing right, drinking water, eating right and going to bed by 10:30 PM. Your body wants to exercise naturally.*

*In my early 20s, all I believed in was cardio. So I did 18 years of cardio-only exercises, like step, kick boxing, spinning, running ... you name it. However it didn't give me the body I wanted. Accompanied by chronic dehydration, poor nutrition and an unhealthy sleep-wake cycle, I was 28 pounds overweight when I turned 40. I then became a personal trainer and started regular weight training at the age of 40, while reducing my cardio to no more than 30 minutes at a time. At the same time, I started drinking more water, going to bed by 10:30 PM, cutting back sugar and other processed foods. In 6 months, I lost 15 pounds. And I lost another 10 pounds within a year.*

*Just at the time I felt I knew it all, in late 2008 and 2009, a bad fall, stress, over-training, plus poor posture, and stiff hip and shoulder joints, all put me through a painful a year and a half experience with a frozen shoulder. I gained 10 lbs. with it. I had to question and rethink everything about the way I exercised. It led me to intensive training with Paul Chek and the C.H.E.K Institute on Corrective Holistic Exercise Kinesiology and the Holistic Lifestyle Coaching program. Using the principles I learned, I healed my right shoulder and lost that 10 lbs. I have maintained my well-being, body weight and fat percentage ever since. The exercise formula I apply every day is:*

**Posture - Stability/Mobility - Strength - Power**

# 6

## *Posture Makes Perfect*

I did quite a bit of heavy weight lifting without any awareness of my poor posture until I got a frozen shoulder in 2008. For a year and a half, I was in pain almost every day and night. Once I started doing posture corrective exercises, like prone cobra, and started stretching my tight chest muscles, strengthening my weak back muscles, as well as working on my emotional challenges, I was able to freely move my right shoulder again.

Good posture keeps muscles in balance and the body in alignment, allowing minimum energy expenditure and optimal efficiency. While poor posture can result in certain muscles tightening up or shortening while others lengthening or become weak, leading to spinal and joint dysfunction and chronic pain. There is static posture and dynamic posture. Static posture refers to the alignment of the body when sitting or standing; dynamic posture refers to the alignment of the body when moving or exercising.

Posture is a daily habit. When you are not aware of it day by day, year after year, it can cause some serious dysfunction and chronic pain. However, it can be retrained by corrective exercises and daily awareness.

## *What Bad Posture Can Cost You*

Poor posture:

» Disturbs optimal breathing patterns. When slumped over, the lungs have less room to contract and inflate, therefore, decreasing their capacity to obtain the maximum amount of oxygen needed.
» Interferes with optimal circulation around joints resulting in waste product build-up and inflammation.
» Carries a high risk for injuries. Many athletes participating in overhead sports with poor posture, like baseball players, are at risk of traumatic or degenerative injuries to the shoulder girdle.
» Carries a high risk of chronic pain in the neck, shoulders, and lower back.

It is impossible to start an exercise program without addressing and correcting posture issues.

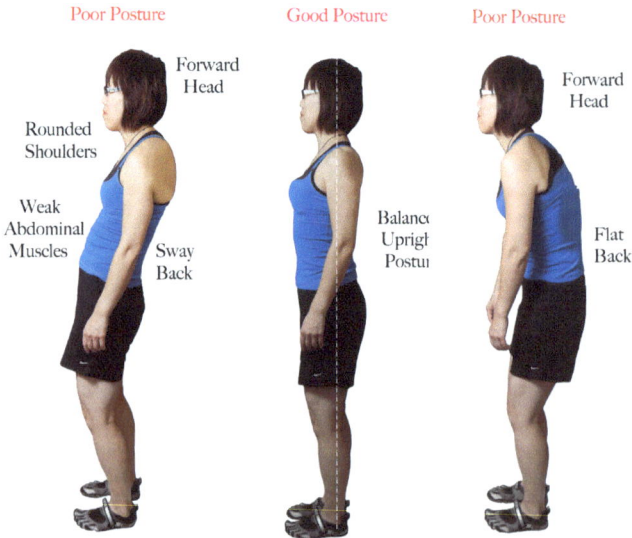

## *Two Types of Poor Posture*

There are two commonly seen poor posture alignments: upper cross syndrome and lower cross syndrome.

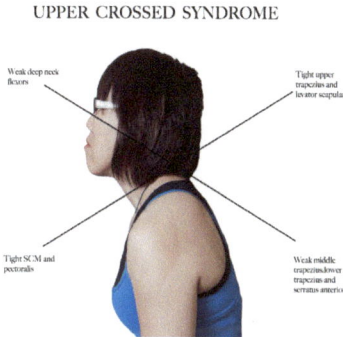

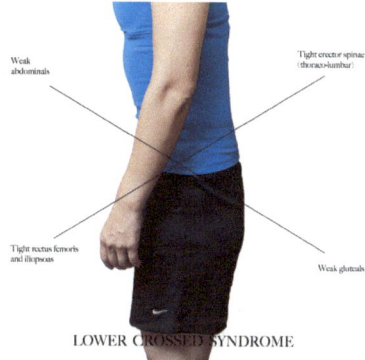

UPPER CROSSED SYNDROME

Weak deep neck flexors

Tight upper trapezius and levator scapular

Tight SCM and pectorals

Weak middle trapezius,lower trapezius and serratus anterior

Weak abdominals

Tight erector spinae (thoraco-lumbar)

Tight rectus femoris and iliopsoas

Weak gluteals

LOWER CROSSED SYNDROME

| Upper Cross Syndrome | Lower Cross Syndrome |
|---|---|
| **Muscle imbalances:**<br>» weak (or long): deep neck flexors; lower trapezius and serratus anterior<br>» tight (or short): upper trapezius and levator scapulae; pectorals | **Muscle imbalances:**<br>» weak (or long): lower abdominals; gluteal muscles<br>» tight (or short): erector spinae (lower back); hip flexors |
| **Posture changes:**<br>» forward head posture<br>» increased lordosis and thoracic kyphosis<br>» elevated and pronated shoulders<br>» rotation or abduction and swinging of the scapulae<br>(Janda, 1988) | **Posture changes:**<br>» anterior pelvic tilt<br>» increased lumber lordosis<br>» lateral lumber shift<br>» lateral leg rotation<br>» knee hyperextension<br>(Janda, 1987) |
| **Predictions of injuries:**<br>» upper back and neck pain<br>» headaches<br>» rotator cuff injury<br>» cervical disc radiculopathy<br>» jaw pain<br>(Dr. Astrid Trim, 2006) | **Predictions of injuries:**<br>» lower back pain<br>» sciatica<br>» disc injury<br>» knee pain<br>» hip pain<br>(Dr. Astrid Trim, 2006) |

## *Tips to Maintain Good Posture*

1. When sitting, sit as tall as you can; tilt your pelvis forward pulling your back in; lift your chest up and forward; keep your chin tucked in; gently pull your shoulders down and back.

2. Take a break every 90 minutes and stretch for 3 minutes.

3. When standing, lift your chest up and forward; keep your chin tucked in; gently pull your shoulders down and back; tilt your pelvis to neutral.

4. When driving, tilt your rear mirror and side mirrors 1 inch higher, so you are forced to sit tall to drive.

## *Posture Corrective Exercises and Key Stretches*

(Love Your Body, Love Yourself Exercise DVD, in which you can find all exercises in this book will be available at www.amazon.com and www.wisdomfitbyoprae.com soon.)

### 1. Prone cobra

**Set up:**
» Lay prone on the floor, arms on sides.

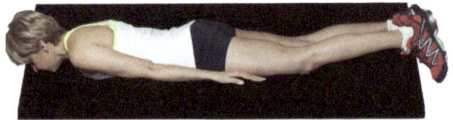

**Start:**
» Inhale and extend thoracic spine while outer rotate (supinate) arms.
» Keep hips and feet on floor.
» Repeat 12-15 times.

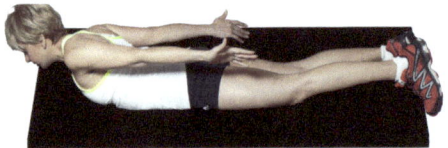

## 2. Upper abdominal stretch on an exercise ball

If you experience any dizziness, please stop performing this stretch.

### Set up:
» Perform this on a non-slip surface.

### Start:
» Sit on the ball, walk your legs out and slowly lie on top of the ball.
» Extend your arms over your head.
» Slowly straighten your legs.
» Breath gently and hold for 60 seconds.

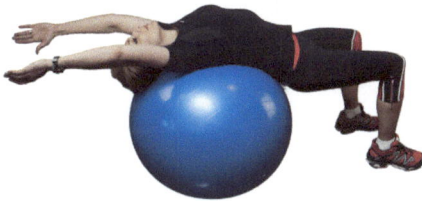

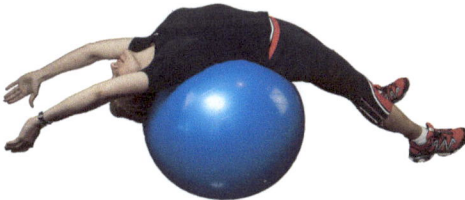

### 3. Hip flexor stretch series

This series of stretch are performed with breathes, also called Stretch Waves (Ann Frederick and Chris Frederick, *Stretch to Win*). They focus on opening up different fascial lines with breathing.

**Set up:**
» From standing, kneel in a lunge position with the right leg back.

**Start:**
**I. Basic**

» Inhale, keeping the chest lifted.
» Slightly pull in your belly button, exhale and press the right hip forward till you feel a gentle stretch.
» Repeat the stretch wave 10 times.

### II. Front line

» Inhale and reach the right arm upward.
» Slightly pull in your belly button, then exhale, lunging into the stretch wave and maintaining a lifted torso.
» Repeat 10 times.

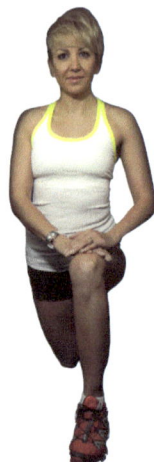

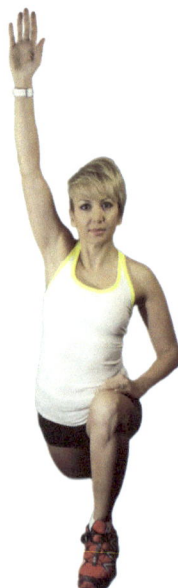

### III. Side line

» From the front line stretch position, inhale and lean the body over to the left side.
» As you exhale into the stretch, slightly push the right hip outward. Inhale as you release.
» Repeat 10 times.

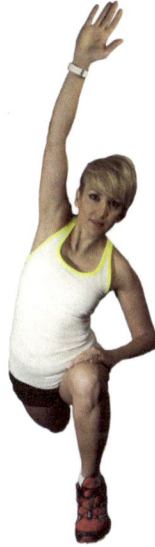

### IV. Rotate torso

» From the leaning position, exhale and rotate the torso by turning the chest upward. Reach the right hand upward and turn the palm up to the ceiling.
» Repeat 10 times.

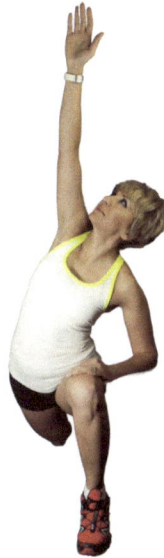

## 4. Wall lean

### Set up:
» Feet should be shoulder-width apart.
» Head, shoulders, back and hips against a wall.

### Start:
» Shift pelvis off the wall while holding neutral spinal alignment.
» Gentle push back of your head into the wall, and straighten your legs, so your hips are off the wall.

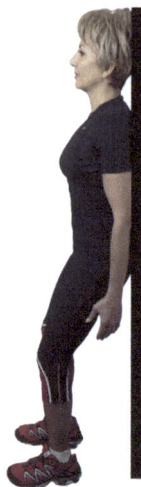

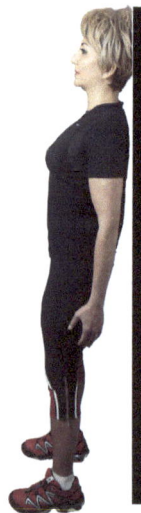

## 5. Lateral neck and levator scapulae

**Set up:**

» Standing upright, place one hand on the top of opposite side of your head.

**Start:**

» Exhale and slowly bend the neck into side flexion; release the stretch while you inhale and repeat the stretch as you exhale.

» To increase the stretch, drop opposite hand and shoulder down to the floor.

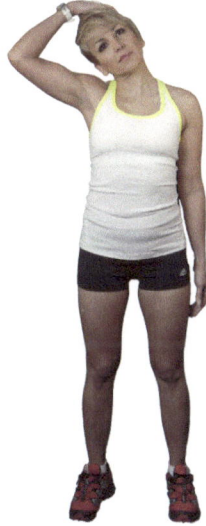

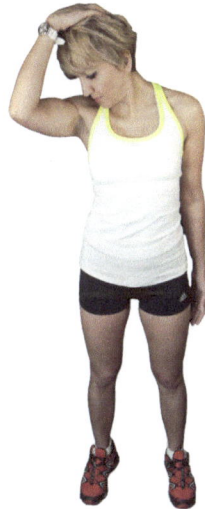

» To add a rotation, rotate the head downward so the eyes are looking toward your underarm.

» Exhale and move the hands back to the top of the head and increase the forward neck bend.

» To increase the stretch, drop opposite hand and shoulder down to the floor.

## 6. Chest stretch on an exercise ball

### I. Pectorals major: (large chest muscle)

**Set up:**
- » Kneel, place your forearm on an exercise ball.
- » Place the other hand on the floor directly beneath the shoulder.
- » Keep your shoulders parallel to the floor

**Start:**
- » Exhale slowly while pressing the arm into the ball and drop your body toward the floor; inhale and release.
- » To increase the stretch, exhale and make a very small circles by directing the ball with arm and shoulder while keeping the tension.

### II. Pectorals minor: (smaller muscle beneath the pectorals major)

**Set up:**
- » Kneel, with one shoulder and elbow at a 90-degree angle on the ball.
- » Place the other hand on the floor directly underneath the shoulder.
- » Keep your torso parallel to the floor.

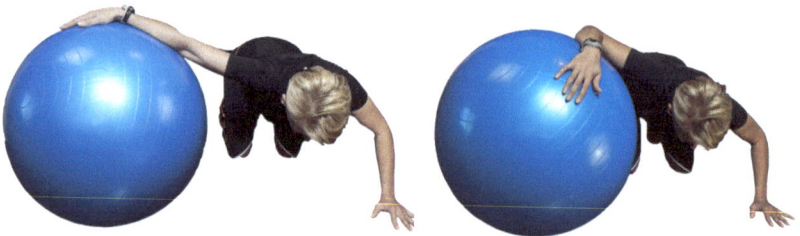

**Start:**

» Exhale, slowly drop your upper body downward while allowing your shoulder blade to move toward your spine.

» To increase the stretch, make very small circles by directing the ball with the shoulder and hand.

## 7. Lower back stretch

**Set up:**

» Lie on your back with knees bent and hands on knees.

**Start:**

» Exhale and pull both knees into your chest.

» Rock back and forth, and side to side while hugging the knees; inhale and release.

» Exhale and drop both knees to one side, keeping shoulders on the floor. Switch to another side.

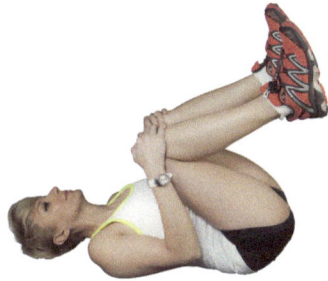

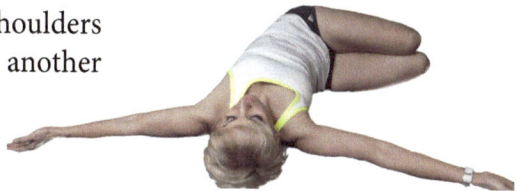

---

················*Take Action*················

*Intentional thought: "I have the best posture. My body is flexible."*

Pick 2-3 stretches that you feel the most, and do them 5 minutes every day.

---

# 7

## *Protect Yourself from Injuries: Stability and Mobility*

### *Why Am I Injured?*

Workout related injuries become widespead, especially in the over 40 population. Common workout injuries include:

» Muscle pull and strain.
» Sprained ankles.
» Shoulder injuries.
» Knee injuries.
» Low back injuries.
» Shin splints.
» Tendinitis.

People usually say "I didn't stretch enough before workout", or "I didn't warm up before". Are stretching and warming up the only ways to prevent workout injuries? They certainly are at superficial level, but not exactly the root cause of injuries.

The real truth is Joint Dysfunction in terms of stability and mobility causes workout injuries. Problems with one joint usually shows up as pain in the joint above or below it. For example an immobile ankle makes unstable knee and may causes knee injury.

**Joint Stability:** The ability to resist movement at a joint from an outside force.

**Joint Mobility:** The ability to move a joint through its full anatomical and available range of motion.

## Joint - By - Joint Approach

Gray Cook, author of *Athletic Body in Balance*, founder of Functional Movement Screening, an Orthopedic and Sports Physical Therapist, developed an easy to understand "Joint - by - Joint" approach. The human body's joints alternate between mobility and stability.

| Joint | Primary Need |
|---|---|
| Ankle | Mobility (sagittal) |
| Knee | Stability |
| Hip | Mobility  (multi-plane) |
| Lumbar Spine | Stability |
| Thoracic Spine | Mobility |
| Scapula | Stability |
| Shoulder | Mobility |

Explained by Michael Boyle (www.graycookmovement com/?p=118) "Loss of function in the joint below - in the case of the lumbar spine, it's the hips - seems to affect the joint or joints above. In another words, if the hips can't move, the lumbar spine will. The problem is the hips are designed for mobility, and the lumbar spine for stability. When the intended mobile joint become immobile, the stable joint is forced to move as compensation, becoming less stable and subsequently painful". In short, immobile hips can cause low back pain.

Keep in mind:

» A loss in ankle mobility may cause knee pain.
» A loss hip mobility may cause low back pain.
» A loss of thoracic mobility may cause neck and shoulder pain, or low back pain.

## *Stability and Mobility Exercises*

(Love Your Body, Love Yourself Exercise DVD, in which you can find all exercises in this book will be available at www.amazon.com and www.wisdomfitbyoprae.com soon.)

## 1. Neck shoulder and upper spine integration (mobility)

**Set up:**
- » Lay on your side with a foam roller, or a towel just big enough to maintain good neck alignment, placed under your head. Your neck should be parallel with the floor.
- » Place your arms out in front and on top of each other.

**Start:**
- » Inhale as you slide the top hand across the bottom arm and your upper body.
- » Exhale as you return, sliding as far forward as you comfortably can, allowing your top hand and wrist to glide over your bottom hand.
- » Do 10 - 20 repetitions on each side.

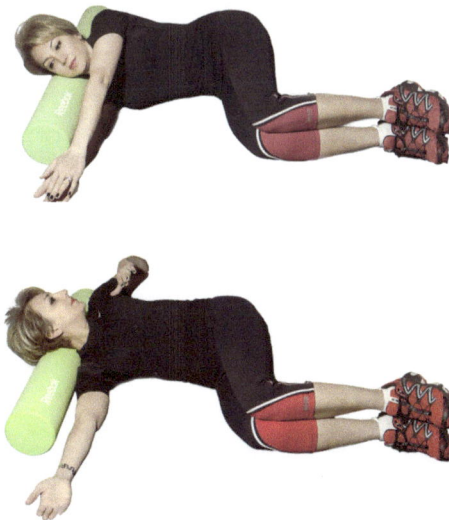

## 2. Trunk rotation (mobility)

### Set up:
» Lay on your back with knees bent 90 degrees, and arms out on the floor.

### Start:
» Exhale and drop both knees to one side, and keep shoulders on the floor.
» Inhale and move back both knees to center. Exhale and drop knees to the other side.

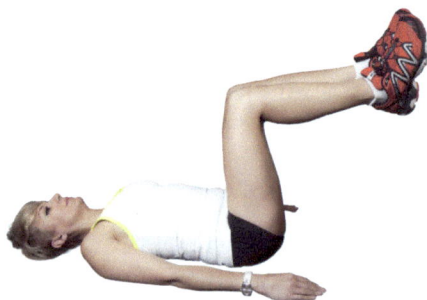

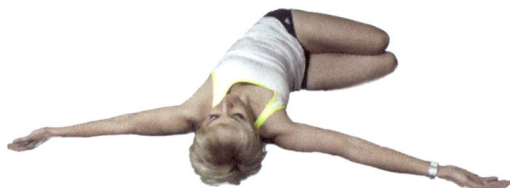

## 3. Thoracic mobilization (mobility)

### Set up:
» Hold your arms straight out to the side, stay relaxed and breathe through your nose naturally.
» Turn your right arm up and left arm down.

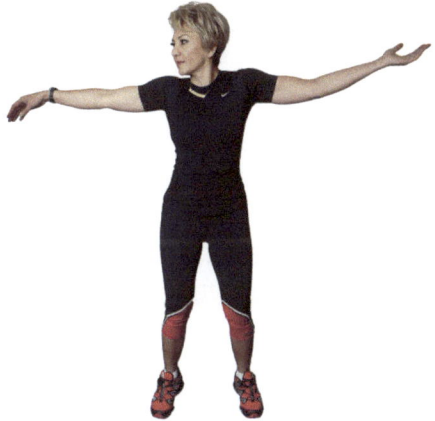

### Start:
» As you look down the left arm, slightly contract the right arm as you turn the palm up and inhale at the same time.
» Exhale and turn your head to the other side and reverse arm positions, repeating the same on the opposite side.
» Do 10 repetitions on each side.

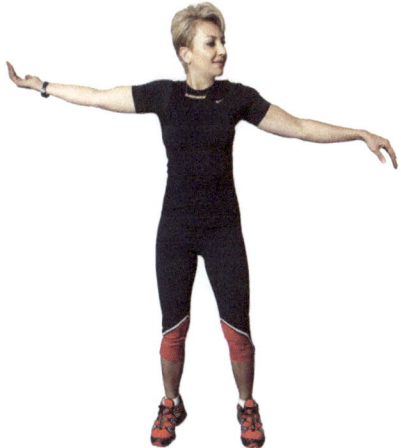

## 4. Hip extension series I, II, III (stability)

### I. Basic

**Set up:**
» Lay on your back with arms placed comfortably on your sides. Your feet are on the floor with knees bent.

**Start:**
» Exhale while lifting your hips up in alignment with your knees and shoulders.
» Inhale while returning your hips to the floor. Exhale and repeat the same movement.
» Do 15 - 20 repetitions.

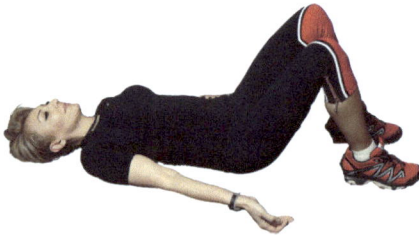

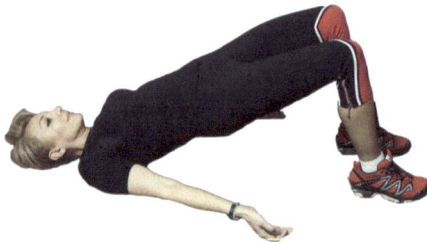

## II. Single leg

» Lift your hips with one leg on the air and the other foot on the floor.
» Do 10-12 repetitions on each side.

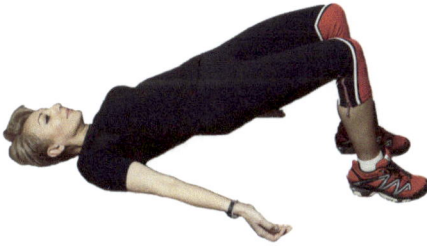

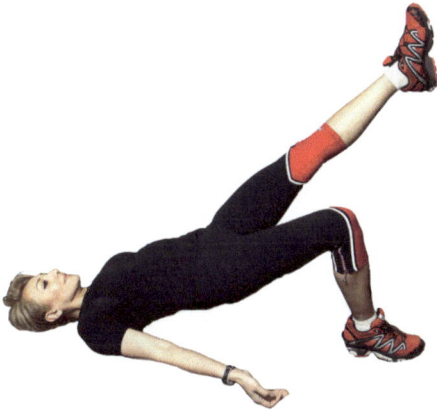

## III. With an exercise ball

**Set up:**
- » Lay on an exercise ball with head and shoulders supported by the the ball. Knees are bent 90 degrees.

**Start:**
- » Exhale and drop your hips vertically without moving the ball.
- » Inhale while pushing your legs through your heels and extend your hips up, parallel to the floor. Maintain 90 degree with knees.

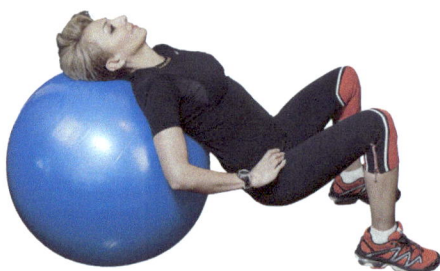

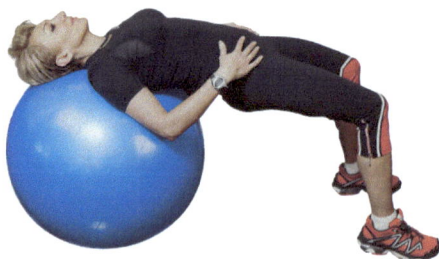

## 5. Horse stance (stability)

**Set up:**
- » Both your hands and knees are on the floor with 90 degrees to hips, knees, and shoulders.
- » Maintain neutral spinal alignment (head - shoulder girdle - hips in one line).

**Start:**
- » Exhale, gently pull your belly button towards to your spine, and raise your left leg parallel to the floor, then lift your right arm 45 degree angle, with an option of the thumb pointing up.
- » Inhale and return to starting position.
- » Repeat each side 10 - 15 repetitions.

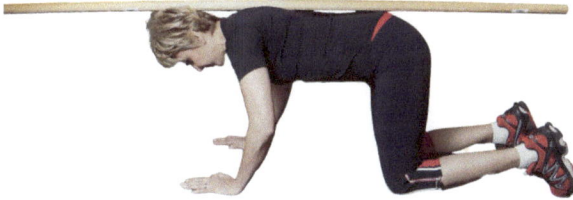

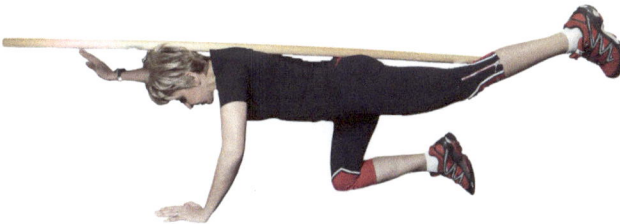

## 6. Supine lateral ball roll (stability)

### Set up:
» Lay supine on an exercise ball - head and shoulders are supported by the ball while maintaining a neutral alignment.
» Palms up with a dowel rod across the chest.
» Hold pelvis level - 90 degrees at knees with weight on the heels.

### Start:
» Laterally shift over ball while keeping your torso parallel to the floor. Hold for 5 - 10 seconds.
» Alternate sides.
» Do 12 - 20 repetitions.

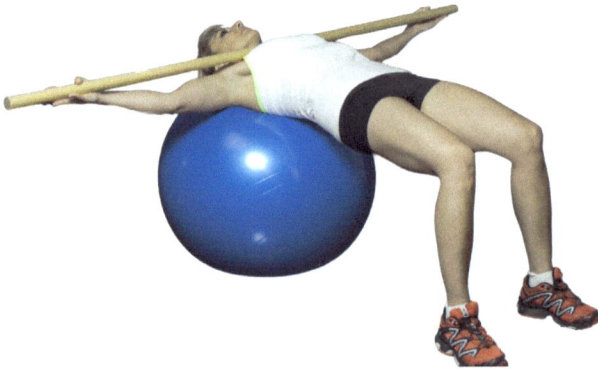

## 7. Single leg standing series I, II, III (stability)

### I. Single leg stands on the floor

**Set up:**
» Stand with feet comfortable and knees slightly bent. Breathe naturally.

**Start:**
» Ground one foot. Gently pull your belly button towards to your spine, and slowly lift the other foot off floor without rotating or lifting your hips.
» Breathe naturally and hold as long as you can.
» Alternate sides.
» Hold for 2 - 3 minutes on each side.

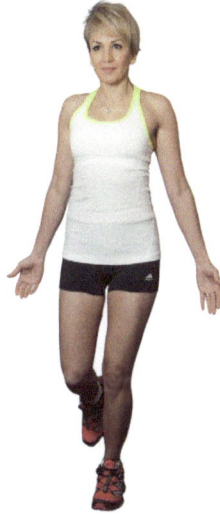

### II. Both feet on a bosu

» Stand on a bosu with knees slightly bent. Gently pull your belly button towards to your spine, and breathe naturally.
» Hold as long as you can.

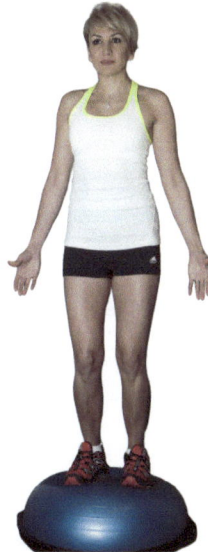

### III. Single leg on a bosu

» Once you are stable with both feet on a bosu, start lifting one foot off the bosu without lifting or rotating your hips.
» Hold as long as you can.
» Switch to the other foot.

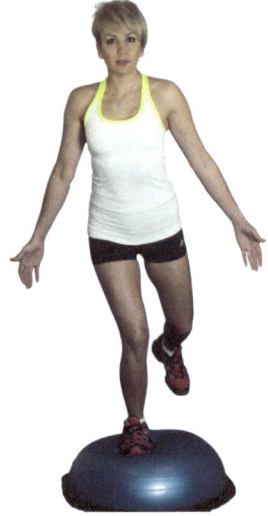

### 8. Full plank series I, II (stability)

**Set up:**

» Facing down, use both your hands and toes to hold your body. Your head, shoulder girdle and hips are in alignment.

**Start:**

### I. Basic

» Slightly pull your belly button towards to your spine, and hold as long as you can.

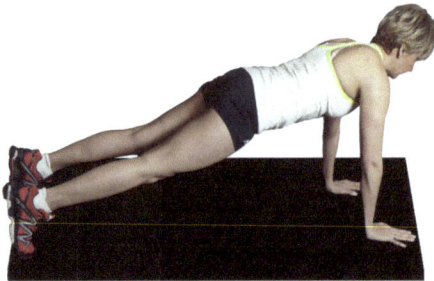

## II. Advanced

» Keep plank position, take one arm off floor and hold it for 3 - 5 seconds.
» Switch sides.
» Do 12 - 20 repetitions.

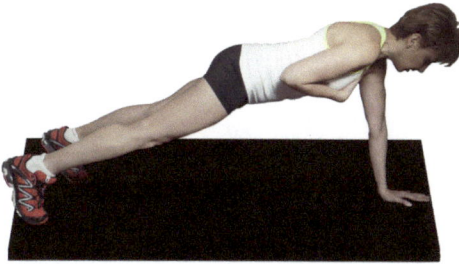

# 8

## Master Primal Movements for Life

### Primal Movement Patterns by Paul Chek

No matter how complicated you think exercising is, the truth is that there are only seven Primal Movement Patterns. (Paul Chek, HHP, NMT). Those primal movement patterns include Squat, Lunge, Push, Pull, Twist, Bend and Gait. Any given movement in life, whether it is throwing a baseball, playing tennis, swinging a golf club, or simply getting out of a car, you are always using a combination of one or more of those 7 primal movement patterns. When I exercise or design an exercise program, the first thing comes to my mind is which movement pattern is going to be involved.

### Squat Exercises

(Love Your Body, Love Yourself Exercise DVD, in which you can find all exercises in this book will be available at www.amazon.com and www.wisdomfitbyoprae.com soon.)

We need to squat to pick up heavy objects like boxes, to sit on the toilet or a chair, or to simply get out of a car.

## 1. Wall squat on an exercise ball

### Set up:
» Place an exercise ball between your lower back and a wall.
» Your feet placed about shoulder-width apart. Your arms are at your sides. Keep your body straight.

### Start:
» Inhale and gently draw your belly button towards your spine. Lower your hips down and back into a squat as if you are sitting on a chair as you exhale.
» Go as low as you comfortably can, then inhale as you return to standing.
» Do 15 - 20 repetitions.

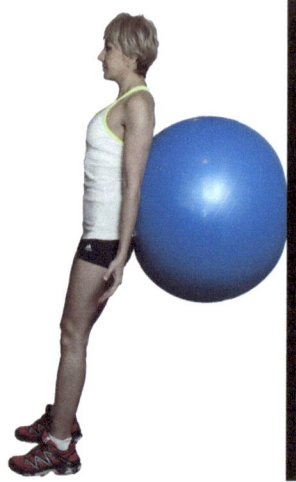

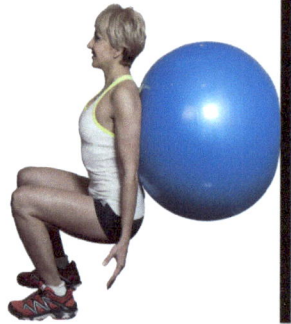

## 2. Squat with a support

### Set up:
» Stand straight with shoulders down and back. Hold a rod in front of your body.

### Start:
» Inhale and gently draw your belly button towards your spine.
» Move your hips down and back into a squat while maintaining a neutral spine as you exhale.
» Inhale and return to standing position.
» Repeat 20 times.

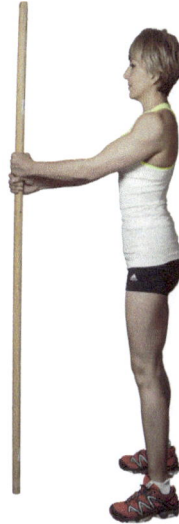

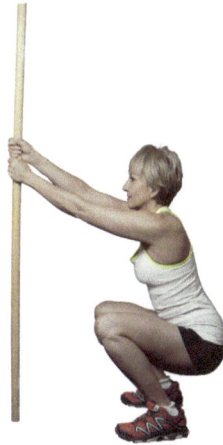

## 3. Kettlebell squat

### Set up:
» Take a comfortable stance and hold two 8kg - 12kg kettlebells at your sides.

### Start:
» Inhale and gently pull your belly button inward.
» Drop your hips down and back as comfortably as you can into a squat while maintaining a neutral spine.
» Exhale as you stand up.
» Do 8 - 12 repetitions.

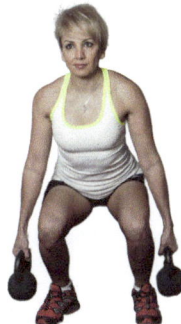

## Lunge Exercises

Lunges are widely seen in sports like in playing squash or tennis. They involve in several joints such as ankles, knees and hips as well as various muscles, such as core muscles, quad / hamstring muscles and gluteus muscles.

### 1. Static lunges with support

**Set up:**
» Have one leg forward and the other back while holding a rod.
» Keep your torso tall and inhale as you gently pull your belly button inward.

**Start:**
» Drop your rear knee down to the floor into a lunge position.
» Return to starting position as you exhale.
» Alternate your legs for 12 - 20 repetitions.

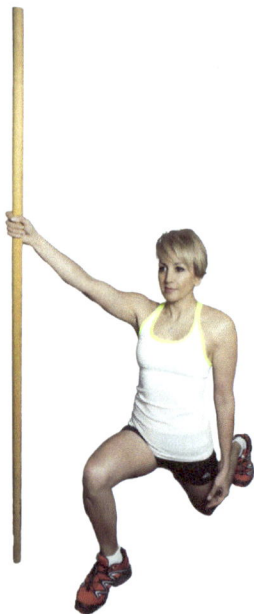

### 2. Walking lunges

**Set up:**
» Begin standing with your feet together and torso tall.

**Start:**
» Gently pull your belly button inward and step forward while dropping your rear knee down to the floor.

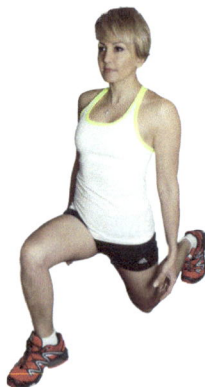

» Alternate your legs and keep moving forward into the lunge position.
» Once you do well with the body weight, you may be able to add two 10 - 15 lbs. of dumbbells.

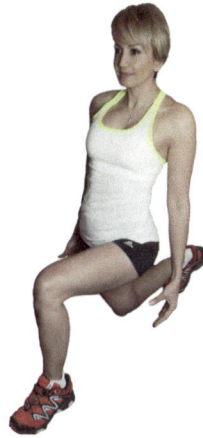

### 3. Lateral lunges

**Set up:**
» Begin standing with feet together and chest open.

**Start:**
» Gently pull your belly button inward and step to the side.
» Keep both feet facing forward and bend the knee you are stepping with. Alternate your legs and repeat.
» Do 20 - 30 repetitions.

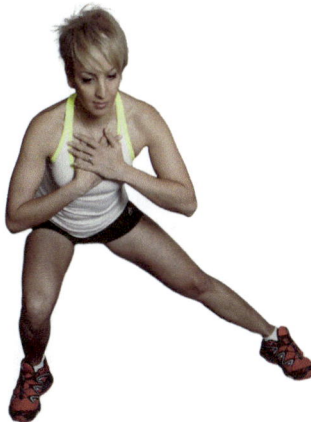

## 4. Overhead lunges

**Set up:**
- » Hold a dumbbell in one hand.
- » Press the weight above your head, and hold it.

**Start:**
- » Gently pull your belly button inward, step forward into a lunge position.
- » Step back, and alternate the other leg. Perform 12 repetitions.
- » Switch weight to the other hand and repeat the same movement for 12 repetitions.

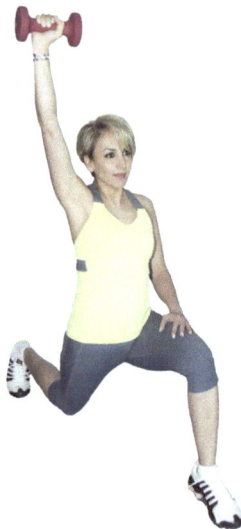

## Bend Exercises

In daily life we bend all the time to tie shoes or pick things up.

## 1. Static bend

**Set up:**
- » Stand and have feet shoulder-width apart.

**Start:**
- » Slightly pull your belly button inward and bend forward. Rest your hands above your knees.
- » Keep your head and spine in a neutral position.
- » Hold the position for 30 - 90 seconds or as long as you can.

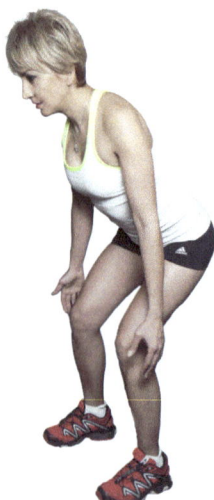

## 2. Sumo deadlift

### Set up:
» Begin with a sumo stance - feet wider than shoulder-width and slightly outward.
» Hold two kettlebells in front of your thighs with one arm pronated and the other arm supinated.

### Start:
» Take a deep diaphragmatic breath and pull your belly button in toward your spine.
» Keep your head, shoulder girdle, and spine in alignment while bending forward until the weight is just above your knees. As the weight passes your knees, use your legs to lower your body down as comfortably as you can.
» Keep your arms close to your body.
» Exhale returning to standing position by pushing your body away from the ground.

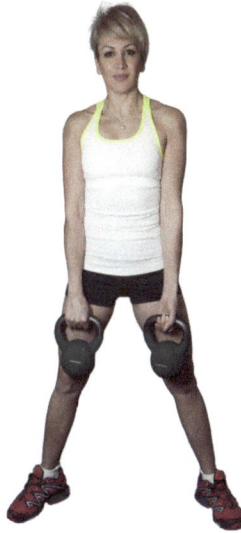

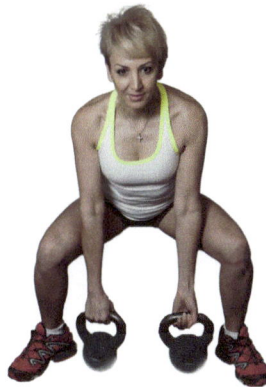

## 3. Single leg deadlift

### Set up:
» Stand with feet slightly open. Hold dumbbells in both hands in front of your body.

### Start:
» Gently pull in your belly button, bend from your hips and lift one leg while keeping your hips parallel to the floor. Keep the weight close to your supporting leg.
» Return to starting position. Perform 10 - 12 repetitions.
» Alternate sides.

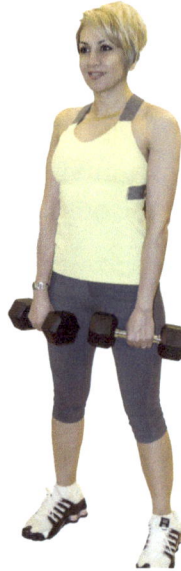

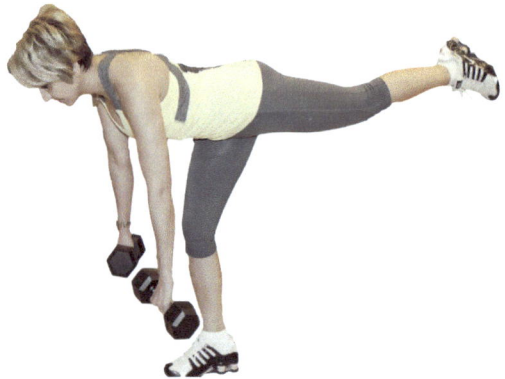

## Twist Exercises

### 1. Supine lateral ball roll

**Set up:**
- » Lay supine on an exercise ball - head and shoulders supported on the apex of the ball to maintain a neutral alignment.
- » Arms out to the sides with palms up and a dowel rod across chest. Feet are wider than shoulder-width.
- » Maintain torso parallel to the floor and 90 degrees at knees.

**Start:**
- » Laterally shift your body over the ball without drop your shoulder and hip. Hold for 3 - 5 seconds.
- » Back to center.
- » Laterally shift your body to the other side and hold for 3 - 5 seconds.
- » Do 12 - 20 repetitions.

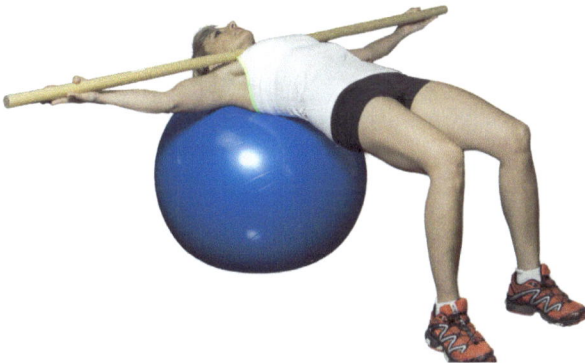

## 2. Cable wood chop

### Set up:
» Facing sideways to a cable column, grasp the handle with two hands, and take a wide stance.
» 70% of your body weight is on the leg that is closer to the cable machine.

### Start:
» Draw your belly button in toward to your spine. Start the movement by bending the other leg, pushing away from the cable machine and rotating your trunk while pulling the handle downward across your body.
» The movement ends when your hands are just above or slightly outside your foot.
» Set up a weight that you can handle doing 12 - 15 repetitions.
» Alternate sides for 12 - 15 repetitions.

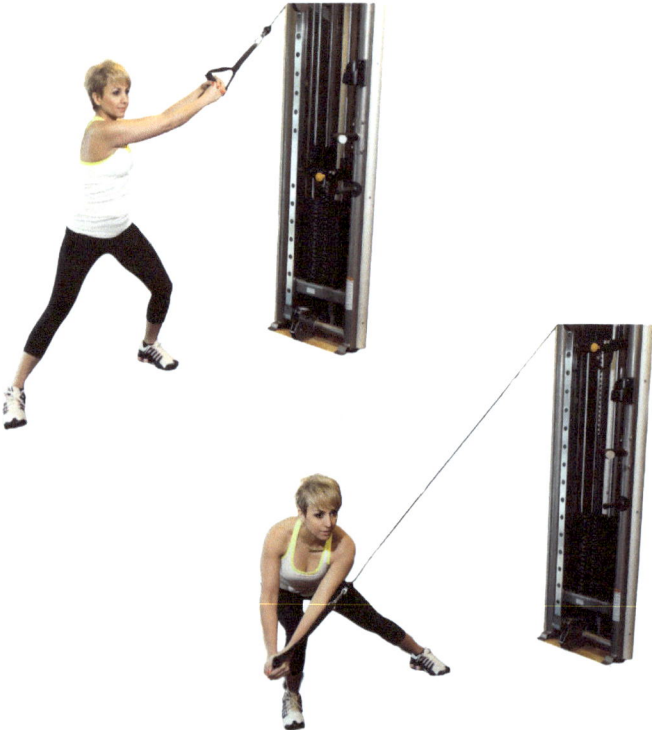

## 3. Russian twist

### Set up:
» Lay your head, shoulders and upper back on an exercise ball. Raise arms up in front of your chest, and palm to palm.
» Lift your hips up so you maintain your torso parallel to the floor.

### Start:
» Place your tongue on the roof of your mouth.
» Rotate the ball under you, going from side - to - side.
» Do not drop your hips.
» Do 20 - 30 repetitions.

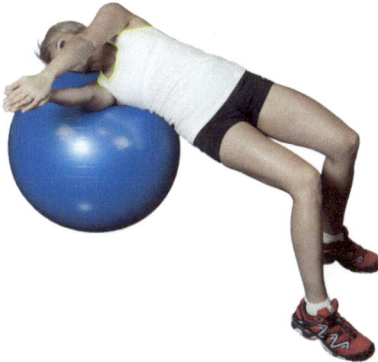

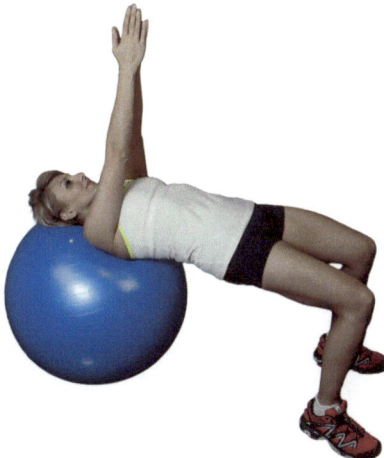

# Push Exercises

## 1. Partial push up

### Set up:
» Place two hands on a bench wider than shoulder-width.
» Arms are at shoulder level.

### Start:
» Draw your belly button in, keep your head, shoulder girdle and spine in alignment, bend your elbows, and take the body towards the bench.
» Exhale and return to starting position without losing your alignment.
» Do 10 - 20 repetitions.

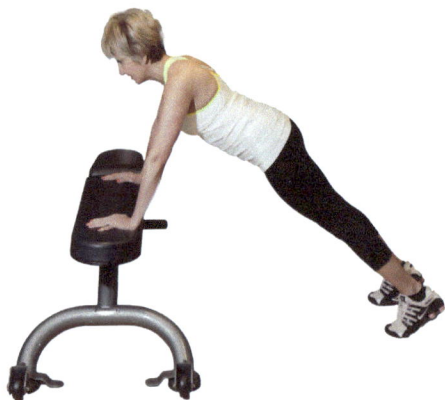

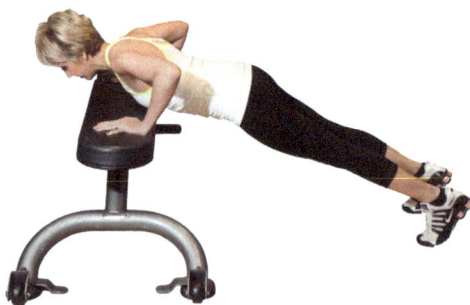

## 2. Push up on floor

(Follow the same instructions in the "partial push up" exercise above except you are going to perform on the floor.)

**Set up:**
  » Place two hands on a floor wider than shoulder-width.
  » Arms are at shoulder level.

**Start:**
  » Draw your belly button in, keep your head, shoulder girdle and spine in alignment, bend your elbows, and take the body towards the floor.
  » Exhale and return to starting position without losing your alignment.
  » Do 10 - 20 repetitions.

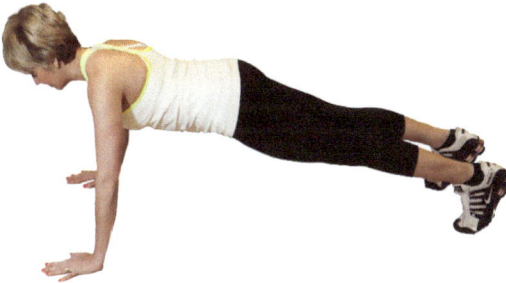

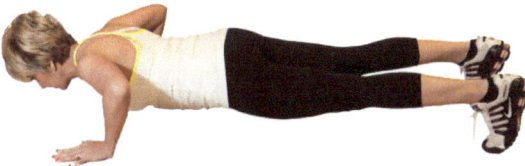

## 3. Single arm cable push

**Set up:**
» Face away from a cable machine that has been adjusted to shoulder height.
» Grab the cable handle using the arm on the same side as the rear leg.
» Keep both knees bent.

**Start:**
» Gently draw your belly button in and move your body weight to the front leg while pushing the side with cable handle forward.
» Return to starting position.
» Do 10 - 15 repetitions on each side.

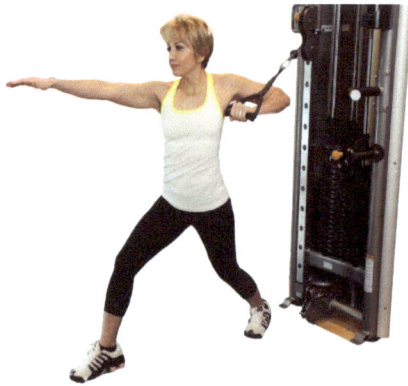

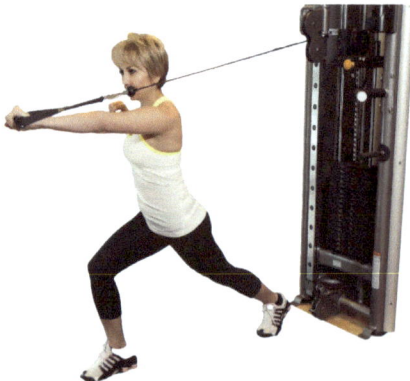

# Pull Exercises

## 1. Single arm bend over row

**Set up:**
- » Take a split stance with both knees bent.
- » Hold a weight (kettlebell) on the same arm as your rear leg.
- » Lean forward with your head, shoulder girdle and back in alignment.

**Start:**
- » Gently pull your belly button in toward to your spine.
- » Pull your arm back while bending your elbow.
- » Do 8 - 12 repetitions.

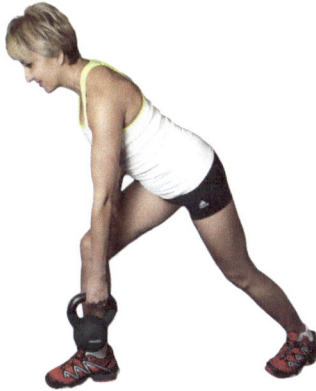

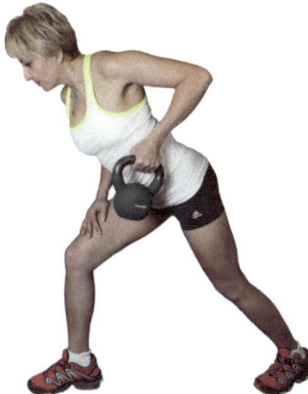

## 2. Single arm cable pull

**Set up:**
- » Stand facing a cable machine that has been adjusted higher.
- » Take a split stance with one leg forward and the other back. Keep knees softly bent.
- » Grab the cable handle and use the same arm as your rear leg.

**Start:**
- » Gently pull your belly button in and initiate the the movement by transferring your body weight to the rear leg while pulling the cable toward your shoulder.
- » Return to start position and do 8 - 12 repetitions. If you feel you still can do more after 12 repetitions, add more weights.

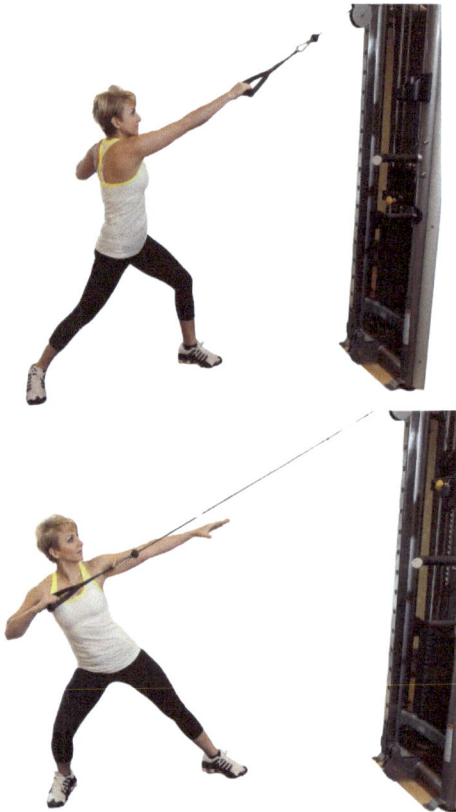

### 3. Pull-up with two Equalizer bars

**Set up:**
- » Lying between two Equalizers with both hands holding on top of the bars, with knees bent.
- » Keep arms 90 degrees to shoulders.

**Start:**
- » Gently pull your belly button in toward your spine, and pull your body up while bending your elbows.
- » Keep your hips in alignment with your head and spine.
- » Do as many as you can without losing your form.

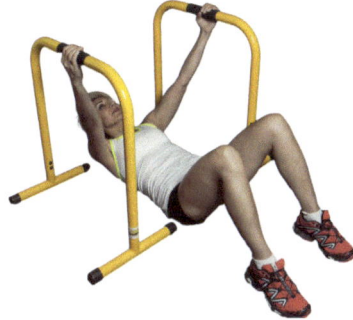

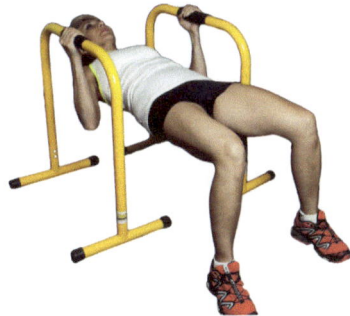

---

························*Take Action*························

*Intentional Thought: "It is easy and fun to exercise."*

1. Have a Squat day by doing 2 - 3 squat exercises, 12 - 20 repetitions, and 2 - 3 sets.

2. Pick 3- 4 exercises from Lunge pattern and Twist pattern and make a circuit workout of 2 - 3 sets.

# 9

## *Less Is More*

### *The Dangers of Over-Training*

There are many benefits of exercising regularly, such as losing weight, strengthening the heart, supporting joints, improving energy, improving mental health, living longer, on and on. However, too much exercise is just as bad as no exercise at all.

My friend Kim and her husband, Vito, have owned All Canadian Martial Arts center since 1989. Believing in "No Pain, No Gain", and following the disciplinary martial art principle of getting through whatever is in the way - whether it is pain, injuries or sickness, she has been pushing herself over the limit. On top of teaching classes and doing her own intensive martial art training, she has been religiously doing her cardio every day for 10 years. After she turned 40, she started to feel her legs were heavier after her workout; she felt tired all the time; and it was taking her 3 times longer to recover from training. When I told her about Less is More, she didn't believe me at first, however she listened and tried to change her exercise routine. She only focused on her martial art training, and completely cut out cardio workouts for 2 years. Instead of cardio, she did regular yoga. Every time I met her for coffee, she told me how much better she felt - she had more energy, with less pain in her shoulders and

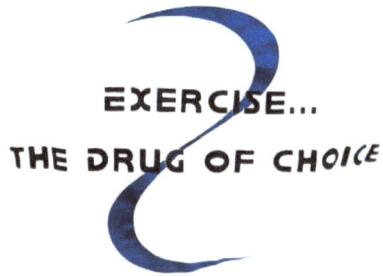

**EXERCISE...**
**THE DRUG OF CHOICE**

neck, and was experiencing a quicker recovery. Now she only does cardio 2-3 times a week for 20 minutes. That is about 60 minutes each week, compared to 45 minutes every day for 5 days, which is 225 minutes of cardio training per week. She is able to manage her body weight, muscle tone and level of strength. She is now a true believer of LESS IS MORE.

Signs of over-training:

» Increase in morning resting heart rate.
» Chronic fatigue.
» Frequent cold or other conditions caused by weakened immune system.
» Recurrent or prolonged injuries.
» Decreased performance - getting weaker and slower.
» Rapid muscle loss, not fat loss.

### Work In or Work Out?

My client, Terry, is a very active 65 year old female. She is a seasonal competitive golfer and tennis player. On top of that she is finishing her master's degree in history at the University of Toronto. She came to my session one day in recovery from almost one week of suffering from a cold, sore muscles and low energy. I did 20 minutes of fascial stretch therapy on her hips, lower back, and shoulders on a massage table at first. Then we did 3 sets of breathing squats, breathing hip extensions on an exercise ball, breathing reverse low back extensions on the ball and very low weight cable pulls (3 inhale and 3 exhale each way). We finished with stretches. She kept telling me that she hadn't felt this good for an entire week. I explained that I had her just do a WORK IN session instead of a WORK OUT session.

The concept of WORKING IN was first created and used by my mentor, Paul Chek, who is the best at teaching and practicing holistic approach to health and fitness. Contrast this with Working Out exercises which increase heart rate and your energy expenditure, Working In exercises are gentle movements with full breaths that help restore energy without raising your heart rate. Breathing squats, Qi Going, Tai Chi, gentle yoga poses and stretches are examples of Working In exercises.

Do not spend more energy than you have. Work with your natural energy flow rather than energy derived from stimulants like coffee, sugar or Red Bull. Pick the right exercises for you on a day-to-day basis and this will have a therapeutic effect on your weight loss, help you build muscles and maintain high level of energy, health and well-being.

Depending on how busy I am and how much energy I have, I choose different types of exercises (Working In or Working Out) with different intensities, repetitions and sets. This helps my body maintain balance of growth and repair. For example, if I have 6 clients in a day, I do more Working In exercises, such as mobilizing, breathing, and stretching to maintain high level of energy and mental focus, and only 10-15 minutes of Working Out exercise, such as front squat and lunges at a higher intensity in shorter time. On the other hand, if I have a light work-day, I will do 45 minutes Working Out exercises using more challenging and energy-demanding movements.

····················································*Take Action*····················································
*Intentional Thought: "I allow myself to take a rest when it is needed."*

# *Part III*

# The Formula of Success

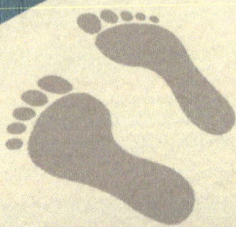

# 10

## *The Formula of Success: A-C-M-A-E*

**A-wareness**
**C-ommitment**
**M-entor**
**A-ction**
**E-ducation**

### *Awareness*

The first step in creating what you want is awareness. It comes from within.

Awareness is the ability to perceive, to feel or to be conscious of events, objects or sensory patterns. Your awareness may be raised by a chronic pain you are experiencing, a book you are reading, a workshop you are attending, a conversation you are having with a friend, a lost of a family member or a friend, or by your own frustration.

Having awareness allows you to recognize your thoughts, beliefs, weaknesses, strengths, as well as your eating and lifestyle patterns. Having awareness also allows you to ask powerful questions, like: "Is this the life and body I really want?" "How can I change?"

Awareness is the first step in changing. It leads to a commitment.

## *Commitment*

Commitment is not only a promise to yourself, it is also a strong desire to do whatever it takes. A committed person takes responsibility for the outcome. She/he is ready to take an action. A committed person doesn't make excuses, she/he makes things happen.

Commitment is the second step in building the body and creating the life you desire.

## *Mentor*

To this day, what has helped me the most is that I always have had a mentor in the area that I felt I needed to grow and improve. 8 years ago when I was struggling the most with my health and exercise regimen, I started to learn from Paul Chek, author of *How to Eat Move and Be Healthy* and founder of C.H.E.K Institute and PPS Success Mastery Program. His system and resources helped me to see immediate results and saved me a lot of energy and saved me time, compared to doing everything on my own.

When I became aware that my old beliefs about myself and my life no longer were working, I started following Luise Hay's work as well as other Hay House authors, like Dr. Wynn Dyer, Dr. Bruce Lipton and more. I attended *I CAN DO IT* conferences and took online courses. All these made a big difference in just a few years.

When I realized financial balance was an important part of my well-being, I found T. Harv Eker, author of *The Secret of Millionaire Mind* and founder of Peak Potential. Going to his 3-day *Millionaire Mind Intensive* training completely opened my eyes to a whole new future of financial freedom, one that we all deserve. It has been a part of my life's journey ever since.

When there was a voice inside me telling me that I wanted to share my knowledge and experience with like-minded people, and to help people over age 40 stop struggling, Raymond Aaron, author of numerous New York Times best-selling books, including *Chicken Soup for the Canadian Soul*, showed up in my life. Through his 10-10-10 writing program, I was guided step by step to write and publish my first book, which you are now reading.

Mentors have been there and have done it. She or he has first hand experience, the knowledge, the resources and a system that is tested, implemented and proven to be successful. So you don't need to make similar mistakes and figure out everything for yourself, which is ineffective and time-consuming. My advice to you is not to listen to your friends or family, they don't know any more than you. Instead find a mentor who is successful in the area you need to work on. Learn the system and put it into practice every day. Believe me, there is always the right teacher waiting for you when you start looking.

## *Action*

You can have the best teacher, coach, or mentor, but no one can do it for you. It is your consistent and conscious action which will produce the result you desire and deserve. It is your life and your body. DO IT FOR YOURSELF.

Dream big, but start small. Always start one step at a time. Do it every day till it becomes your subconscious habit. Then go for another one. The good news is that research shows, you can build a new habit in as little as 21 days. When I decided to limit my sugar and bread, I started out by cutting my intake to half. After a few months, I had it every other day, then every 2 days, every 3 days, finally once a week, once every two weeks, once a month... After one year I was surprised at how easy it had been to eliminate them. I wasn't craving sugar or bread any more.

Over 10 years I changed so many habits without feeling I have done that much.

## *Education*

In order to stay on the right track and become more successful, it is important to continue to educate yourself on a regular basis. A new level of awareness and consciousness can now be vividly in your mind as a result of education. You will now come up with new commitments and find the right mentor to guide you into putting them in action. It is like taking stairs. In order to reach the highest floor, you have to keep climbing, repeating the same steps: A-C-M-A-E.

I am constantly learning new things every week: listening to presentations and podcasts from reputable resources; reading new articles and books; going to seminars, events and conferences. It is so much fun to learn things that support my health, fitness as well as my spirit and finances. When I stop learning, I start dying.

## *Slow Pace Wins the Game*

> *"A journey of a thousand miles*
> *must first begin with a single step."*
> *- Lao Tzu, 604 - 531 BC,*
> *The Tao Te Ching, 64 verse*

..............................................

Patience is the key to success. Unfortunately we are living in a fast pace world in which everyone wants a magic pill or quick fix. However life does not work that way. Life is running according to your daily choices and habits. Focusing on making the right choices and building the right habits every day will take you where you want to go. So relax and enjoy your journey.

When I decided to write this book, I made a plan of writing 300 words every day or 1500 words a week. 10 months later I had reached the last chapter, had written 21,000 words and done all of the illustrations and exercise pictures. I wasn't overwhelmed or stressed. Actually I was enjoying every day writing.

## *Final Thoughts*

*It is never too late to make a change.*

*Life is a journey. Life is an art. Enjoy it step by step, piece by piece, day by day. You are worth it.*

*You are loved and supported.*

# References and Resources

## *Part I*

## 1. Change Your Thoughts, Change Your Body

1. Louise Hay, You Can Heal Your Life, Hay House, Inc., 2004.
2. Bruce Lipton, The Biology of Beliefs, Hay House, Inc., 2005.
3. http://www.youtube.com/watch?v=jjj0xVM4x1I: Documentary The Biology of Beliefs by Bruce Lipton.
4. Cheryl Richardson, The Art of Extreme Self Care, Hay House, Inc., 2009.
5. Marianne Williamson, A Course in Weight Loss, 21 Spiritual Lessons for Surrendering Your Weight Forever, Hay House, Inc., 2010.
6. Dr. Wayne Dyer, Change Your Thought Change Your Life, Hay House, Inc., 2007.
7. www.hayhouseradio.com.

## 2. The Secret to Having Energy

1. Dennis Lewis, The Tao of Natural Breathing, Rodmell Press, 2006.
2. Paul Chek, Workshop, Respiration the Science of Breathing and Movement, C.H.E.K Institute, 2011.
3. Paul Chek, Video: Breathing Basics Part 1: http://www.youtube.com/watch?v=UlJEkHJCMqc.
4. James L. Wilson, N.D., D.C., Ph.D., Adrenal Fatigue - The 21st Century Stress Syndrome, Smart Publications, 2000.

## 3. The Wonder of Weight Loss

1. F. Batmanghelidj, M.D., Your Body's Many Cries for Water, second edition, Global Health Solutions, Inc., 1997.
2. http://drsircus.com/medicine/water/dehydration-3.
3. www.watercure.com.
4. Sherry A. Rogers, M.D., Detoxify or Die, Sandy Key Company, Inc., 2002.

## 4. Transform Your Body Effortlessly with Sleep

1. T.S. Wiley with Bent Formy, Ph.D., Lights Out: Sleep, Sugar and Survival, Pocket Books, 2001.
2. Paul Chek, How to Eat, Move and Be Healthy, C.H.E.K. Institute, 2004.
3. www.sleepfoundation.org.

## 5. 7 Simple Ways of Eating Right for YOU

1. Dr. Weston A. Price, Nutrition and Physical Degeneration, 1930s.
2. Roger J. Williams, Ph.D., Biochemical Individuality, 1956.
3. William Wolcott and Trish Fahey, The Metabolic Typing Diet, Doubleday, 2000.
4. Paul Chek, How to Eat, Move and Be Healthy, C.H.E.K. Institute, 2004.
5. Professor Robert H. Lustig's video lecture: Sugar, the Bitter Truth, http://www.youtube.com/watch?v=dBnniua6-oM.
6. Mary G. Enig, Ph.D., Know Your Fats: The Complete Primer for Understanding the Nutrition of Fat, Oils and Cholesterol, Bethesda Press, 2000.
7. Jeffrey M. Smith, Genetic Roulette: The Documented Health Risks of Genetically Engineered Foods, Yes! Books, 2007.
8. www.responsibletechnology.org.
9. Dr. William Davis, Wheat Belly: Lose the Wheat, Lose the Weight, and Find Your Path Back to Health, Harper Collins Publishers Ltd, 2012.
10. Dr. William Davis, video lecture: Wheat: The UNHealthy Whole Grain, http://www.youtube.com/ watch?v=UbBURnqYVzw.
11. David Perlmutter, M.D. with Kristin Loberg, Grain Brain: The Surprising Truth About Wheat, Carbs, and Sugar - Your Brain's Silent Killers, Little, Brown and Company, 2013.

# Part II

## 6-9

1. Paul Chek, How to Eat, Move and Be Healthy, C.H.E.K. Institute, 2004.
2. Paul Chek, The Golf Biomechanics Manual, 3rd Edition, C.H.E.K. Institute, 2009.
3. Ann Frederick and Chris Frederick, Stretch to Win, Human Kinetics, 2006.
4. Gray Cook's work: www.graycook.com.
5. Paul Chek, C.H.C.K. Exercise Coach course manual, C.H.E.K. Institute, 2009.
6. Paul Chek, C.H.C.K. Practitioner Level One course manual, C.H.E.K. Institute, 2009.